THE SECRET OF SELF-TRANSFORMATION

The Secret of Self-Transformation

A Synthesis of Tantra and Yoga

ROHIT MEHTA

MOTILAL BANARSIDASS PUBLISHERS
PRIVATE LIMITED • DELHI

First Edition: Delhi, 1987
Reprint: Delhi, 1995, 1997, 2000, 2003

© MOTILAL BANARSIDASS PUBLISHERS PRIVATE LIMITED
All Rights Reserved

ISBN: 81-208-0402-3

Also available at:

MOTILAL BANARSIDASS
41 U.A. Bungalow Road, Jawahar Nagar, Delhi 110 007
8 Mahalaxmi Chamber, 22 Bhulabhai Desai Road, Mumbai 400 026
120 Royapettah High Road, Mylapore, Chennai 600 004
236, 9th Main III Block, Jayanagar, Bangalore 560 011
Sanas Plaza, 1302 Baji Rao Road, Pune 411 002
8 Camac Street, Kolkata 700 017
Ashok Rajpath, Patna 800 004
Chowk, Varanasi 221 001

Printed in India
BY JAINENDRA PRAKASH JAIN AT SHRI JAINENDRA PRESS,
A-45 NARAINA, PHASE-I, NEW DELHI 110 028
AND PUBLISHED BY NARENDRA PRAKASH JAIN FOR
MOTILAL BANARSIDASS PUBLISHERS PRIVATE LIMITED,
BUNGALOW ROAD, DELHI 110 007

Introduction

PERHAPS the subtitle of the book will put in greater relief the line adopted in the discussion of the subject—the secret of self-transformation. The main theme is examined in the context of Yoga and Tantra—the two principal spiritual traditions of India. A synthesis between the two is the prime need of our modern scientific and technological civilization. If the modern age is to come out of the morass in which it finds itself, it is urgently necessary that we explore the way of synthesis indicated in this book. Tantra means technique, and Yoga means perception. As one of our eminent scientists, F. Capra says: 'We are in the midst of a crisis of perception.' Yoga represents philosophy—in fact, Yoga is included among the six systems of philosophy discussed in the Hindu thought. And philosophy means *darśana* or perception. Thus, Yoga belongs to the sphere of perception. And Tantra, since it means technique, is essentially concerned with practice. Perception alone is not enough, nor is practice alone sufficient. They must go together. Modern technology has imparted to the present age an element of speed. In fact, speed is one of the main characteristics of the modern age. It is to be seen in all spheres of life's manifestations. But speed has a validity only in the context of direction. Without knowing one's direction, mere speed may land us into strange and even dangerous realms. This is exactly what is happening in the modern world. We have nuclear power, but for what is it to be used? For human destruction, as seems to be the tendency in which its use is moving, or is it to be used for human betterment? If so, what is human betterment? Do we know the direction in which human betterment lies?

Perhaps, we have no time to consider the question of direction, speed alone seems to be sufficient. But this has landed us into dangerous situations. Technology must be associated with right philosophy, for philosophy is the search for direction. And among various schools of philosophy, in the East as well as the West, Yoga is certainly the most relevant to the age in which we live.

Unfortunately, both Tantra and Yoga have become greatly clouded during the passage of time. The present book strives to clear misunderstandings and misconception regarding both Yoga and Tantra. The whole problem of a synthesis between the two has been discussed in the context of the individual, for a transformed individual alone can become a nucleus for fundamental social change. The individual must become a nucleus, not just a centre, for a centre is too static, it is the nucleus which has the dynamic quality. We live in a nuclear age where we have seen what happens when the energy enshrined in a nucleus is released, a nucleus in the realm of matter. If a nucleus of a new consciousness is established, then self-transformation will be done by that nucleus itself.

This nucleus that we are talking about must have both energy as well as vision or direction. The needed energy is within the province of Tantra, while the right direction comes within the realm of Yoga. Yoga without Tantra becomes powerless, just as Tantra without Yoga becomes visionless.

In the synthesis between Yoga and Tantra the indication is for a reunion of psychology and philosophy. Formerly, psychology was a branch of philosophy in the West, it has always been so in the East. But with the rise of science, psychology separated itself from philosophy because of its desire to be recognized as a science. This divorce has caused havoc, for psychology today has lost the vision of philosophy, and philosophy, too, has become a mere intellectual speculation. Philosophy and psychology must once again come together. It is the purpose of this book to suggest their reunion, for only in such reunion can we see the solution of the technological and psychological problems of our age.

In the synthesis of Yoga and Tantra lies the secret of the transformation of the individual, and, of the world as well.

ROHIT MEHTA

Contents

1. The Search for Health

THE PRESENT-DAY civilization is sick, so say many a psychologist and a large number of social philosophers. It is a strange statement in the context of the modern age which has witnessed, and is witnessing, a great increase in the span of human life with the longevity steadily going up. In a period when hygienic and sanitary conditions of towns and cities have considerably improved and when recent developments of medical science have brought under control many incurable diseases, to talk of sickness seems utterly incongruous. And yet it is true that the present civilization is not only sick but dangerously ill. Modern age is becoming more and more health-conscious. Hundreds of people, particularly in the developed countries, rush to centres where newer and newer types of healing practices are advocated. It is needless to say that it is only when men and women are ill that they become more and more health-conscious, and are attracted towards all types of health and healing practices. Yoga practices for health have become quite fashionable. A healthy man is not conscious of health. And so the recent explosion in the field of health and healing devices is clearly indicative of the fact that something is wrong with the patterns of modern life.

We talk very much today about psycho-somatic illnesses as if they are a new variety of illness which has suddenly cropped up, and was unknown in earlier ages. But this is not so, for psychosomatic illnesses have always been there, maybe not in such a virulent form as is witnessed today. We usually make a division between the illnesses of the body and those of the mind. We are very much under the sway of Cartesian thinking, a legacy of Descartes and Newton. This is dialectical thinking or thinking in opposites. It is out of this thinking that there has arisen a mecha-

1

nistic approach to life. Under the spell of this thinking the entire
universe is thought of as a machine, including the human body.
This mechanistic concept still persists, and is very much a part
of our thinking even today in spite of the new developments in
science, particularly physics. And it is this which underlies our
concept of health and illness also even to this day. Dr. Larry
Dossey, in his very fascinating book, *Time, Space and Medicine*,
says:

> The Cartesian formulation led to the view that the body re-
> flected the machine-like characteristics of the universe itself—
> machine-like bodies inhabiting a machine-like world. Disease
> thus arose as a disorder of mechanism. Something went
> awry in the machine.

The question arises : is mechanistic approach tenable in the face
of modern scientific advances? A mechanistic approach is obviously based on fragmentation, breaking up a thing or an event
into its constituent parts. A dissection of reality, according to
this approach, is the only way to understand that reality. The
philosophy of Descartes and the scientific method of Issac Newton arising from it have been the basis of men's thinking for over
three hundred years. According to this, the human body is a mere
collection of parts just as the universe, too, is nothing more than
the assembly of different parts. In this mechanistic approach,
mind and matter are naturally regarded as irreconcilable opposites.
F. Capra in his book, *The Turning Point*, says :

> Descartes' view of living organisms has had a decisive influ-
> ence on the development of life-sciences....The problem is that
> scientists, encouraged by their success in treating living organ-
> isms as machines, tend to believe that they are nothing but
> machines. The adverse consequences of this reductionist
> fallacy have become specially apparent in medicine, where the
> adherence to the Cartesian model of the human body as a
> clockwork has prevented doctors from understanding many of
> today's major illnesses.

The philosophy of mind versus matter, propounded by Descartes, has brought into the realm of perception and understanding much confusion. It has to be remembered that there is, in fact, no dichotomy between mind and matter; they, indeed, are but two aspects of the same phenomenon. They are a unified whole, and, therefore, cannot be isolated. The whole approach of man today in all spheres of life is based on dichotomy, and, therefore, fragmentation. In the universe nothing exists in isolation. Many years ago Sir Arthur Eddington summed up the whole problem in just one sentence when he said : 'The electron vibrates and the whole universe shakes.' Nothing can ever be understood by a process of isolation. It is no exaggeration to say that one cannot understand anything unless one understands everything. But we seem still to be guided by the philosophy of Descartes, not only at the individual level but also at the social or collective level. Descartes said : 'I consider the human body as a machine. My thought compares a sick man and an ill-made clock with my idea of a healthy man and a well-made clock.' Today in all spheres of life there appears to be the sway of the mechanistic approach. Life is regarded as a huge machine, and like all machines it has to be handled part by part. The various departments of life are regarded as separate, one from the other, in almost water-tight compartments. But nothing can exist in isolation, and so by such fragmented approach the livingness of everything that is sought to be understood is lost. With fragmented approach we deal with dead entities, not living ones. In fact, one is reminded of the words of the well-known man of medicine, Alexis Carel, who says : 'Look at the modern man—he wishes to understand the living by dissecting the dead.' That which is living is an integral part of everything else. To isolate anything is to render it dead. This, indeed, is the problem in matters of health and healing.

We are not suggesting that the parts do not exist, and that the condition of the parts is not to be taken into consideration. What we are suggesting is that the parts must be seen in the context and the perspective of the whole. Sri Aurobindo, the great mystic philosopher of modern India, says that one must know the whole before one can understand the part. Ill-health, whether individual or social, arises obviously, because the part is seen as if it exists by itself, isolated from the whole. The economy of life proclaims that prosperity at one level can never come into existence if impoverishment obtains at other levels. Prosperity at one place and impoverishment at the other cannot co-exist. All our economic and social planning is bound to fail, if it is based on isolation and fragmentation. And this applies equally to all so-called spiritual and religious movements also, if they strive to exist and to operate in a state of exclusiveness in their content and process. There has to be an all-inclusive approach or an integrated approach which excludes nothing. This applies as much to bodily health as to scientific investigations or philosophical explorations or to mystical experiences. The essential need of the present age is to move away from a fragmented approach to an integral understanding of man, nature and reality. Unfortunately there is, however, today a tremendous hangover from the intellectual legacy of Descartes and Newton. About this legacy, F. Capra says in his *Tao of Physics* :

> The birth of modern science was preceded and accompanied by a development of philosophical thought which led to an extreme formulation of the spirit-matter dualism. This philosophy appeared in the 17th century in the writings of Rene Descartes who based his views of Nature on a fundamental division into two separate and independent realms—that of mind (*res congitans*) and that of matter (*res extense*). The Cartesian division allowed scientists to treat matter as dead and completely separate from themselves and to see that material world as a multitude of different objects assembled into a huge machine.

In our thinking today, all spheres of life are dominated by this mechanistic approach. It is no exaggeration to say that in this age the mind of man has reached a summit of mathematical and mechanical thinking. There is no wonder that man today seeks answers to all problems of life in terms of mathematical calculations. We live in a computer age, and computer seems to be man's highest achievement. We seem to regard computer as omniscient, capable of giving answers to all questions of life. This mechanistic view of life is based on strict determinism. But, in the context of Heisenberg's Principle of Uncertainty, modern science is today engaged in revising its concepts of causality. We are accustomed to regard all phenomena in terms of cause and effect. But is effect different from cause ? Is there a duality of cause and effect? Today it is the very concept of duality that is being challenged, not so much by philosophical non-dualism but by modern physical science itself. This dualism gave to modern science, during the last more than three centuries, the status of absolute objectivity. The duality of subject and object has not only ruled modern science, it has become the basis of all our thinking irrespective of the department of life in which human intellect functions. However, in the recent advances of modern physics, the separation of the observer from the observed seems meaningless, for, as the scientist John Wheller says, the term observer must be replaced by the word participator. It is being increasingly recognized that there is no observer independent of the act of observation. The observer is an integral part of observation. If that be the case, then the human intellect, which is the observer, can never have an objective view of men and things. The subjectivity of science is becoming more and more recognized in the intellectual world. Now the mind of man functions only in the realm of duality. It is for ever a stranger to the non-dual experience. All knowledge of the mind is relational, it knows a thing in relation to something else. It never knows a thing by itself. And so the dualistic concept in the act of perception must be radically revised.

It is hardly necessary to say that the dualistic approach is the approach of division or fragmentation. Life is a whole and does not lend itself to division. In fargmentation there is a lack of right perception, and without right perception right action is impossible. A right perception does not mean an indifference to the part or the parts. It indicates the perception of the whole in the part itself. As David Bohm, the scientist says, the whole is mysteriously present in the part, even in the tiniest part. The whole is in the part and not away from it. In all cases of ill-health, the part has to be taken into account, but this means that the part must be seen in the context of the whole. And so the philosophy of the whole does not ignore the existence of the part, rather it enables one to see the part in right perspective. But if the whole is in the part, why does not one see it? The question is: how is one to see the whole in the part? In one of the major Upaniṣads, *Īśā Upaniṣad,* it is stated that the whole is whole, even when everything is taken away from it the whole remains the whole. Obviously, the whole refers to the quality of things, and so the whole suffers no diminuation by any quantitative alteration. Thus, the whole is concerned with the quality and not with quantity. A quantitative approach refers to the parts. But the quality resides even in the tiniest part. The mind of man judges all things by measurement. It seeks to measure everything. But in measurement, however exact and precise it may be, the quality escapes. We live today in a civilization which judges everything by measurement. All our values are based on such measurements. Needless to say, in measurement part is regarded as existing by itself. In this approach interrelationship is completely lost sight of. However, today it is isolation and fragmentation that rule the intellectual world. We need remember what modern physics says: you cannot know anything unless you know everything. Anything has no existence apart from everything. Modern scientists tell us that they see only interrelatedness everywhere, not any isolated thing. No doubt, there are parts but they contain the whole. A shift from quantitative to qualitative approach demands a fundamental transformation, not merely in thought but in the very process of thinking. A transformation of thought is easy enough and is going on all the time. But then these altered thoughts arise from the same Cartesian or dialectical thinking. There has to take place a fundamental change from dialectical to integral thinking. But then such radical transformation demands tremendous engergy. Does modern man have that energy ? He is, by and large, an enervated individual. There is today an unprecedented energy crisis, not so much external as internal. Unless human consciousness experiences a release of fresh energy, there is no prospect of man dealing effectively with the crisis that has overtaken human civilization today. How is man to come to the experience of new energy? Can energy be created? If the answer is in the affirmative, the question still is: how is new energy to be created? This is fundamentally the problem of Yoga and Tantra. It has to be remembered that not Tantra alone, but also not Yoga alone. It is in the synthesis of Yoga and Tantra that man can understand the secret of creating new energy, and it is only thus that he can comprehend the secret of transformation.

2. The Energy Crisis

MODERN physical science tells us that energy can neither be created nor destroyed. If so, how can the internal energy crisis facing human beings today be resolved? We have said that the shift from the quantitative to qualitative approach to life demands great energy, for it constitutes a major transformation in the field of consciousness. All transformations, whether structural or functional, need surplus energy, the latter more than the former. From where is the surplus energy to come, if no new energy can be created ? It is true that new energy cannot be created, but energy can be transformed. Such transformation of energy is taking place all the time in nature. The potential energy and the kinetic energy are two principal aspects of energy functioning, and the change over of one from the other is known in the scientific field. While new energy cannot be created, the flow of energy can be handled successfully so that the potential can be made kinetic. When we say, as discussed in the last chapter, that the problem of health or ill-health centres round the question of energy, we suggest that the impediments to the flow of energy can be removed. When this is done, the areas from where impediments have been removed experience a fresh flow of energy. If men experiences ill-health, then it is obviously due to the fact that there exists some blockage in the flow of energy. This applies to the health problems of the individual as also of the society.

Now such blockage of energy operates at various levels, for there are various centres of energy functioning. Energy is, of course, one but it is given different names in accordance with the area of its functioning. However, we are not just now concerned with the various aspects of energy functioning. We shall

8

come to it later in the book. Just at present we are interested in the energy blockage that takes place at the physical or biological level. It is the biological blockage of energy which is the cause of illness seen in life either of the individual of the society.

Now all blockages create divisions and fragmentations. In such fragmentation energy flow is impeded. And so the removal of blockages is most relevant to the approach of wholeness a subject of which we made reference in the last chapter.

We live today in an age of specialization. It is hardly necessary to point out that in specialization a part is sought to be understood in isolation. In every faculty of life, specialization has become the order of the day. We are not suggesting that specialization is not necessary; it is necessary, nay, it is essential. The complexity of life demands such specialization. But if the parts have no existence *per se*, then any understanding of the part or the parts will be devoid of meaning. However, it is being increasingly realized in sphere after sphere of human endeavour that there must be a holistic approach. Wholeness is being accepted in all faculties of human learning. But then what is wholeness? Is wholeness identical with totality? It is quite evident that totality is the sum of the parts. Is wholeness arrived at by totalizing the parts? If it were, then the mechanistic approach would be perfectly valid. Is life a machine? one can dismantle a machine and reassemble the parts for making that machine function effectively. If life were a machine, such dismantling and reassembling would enable one to solve the problems of life. But this approach has not helped us to solve our problems, not even at the level of bodily health. Health is not absence of illness. Even when all symptoms of ill-health are removed, man may not experience the joys of health. Illness is not the accumulation of symptoms. There is something more to health than the removal of symptoms. There have been cases where medical analysis, even the most sophisticated, has not detected any symptom of illness, and yet the man is ill. There is, no doubt, a need for detailed diagnosis, that is, a detailed examination of the parts of the body. But this is not enough, for cne may successfully deal with the part or the parts of the body and yet health may not be restored. Why? This is because the part or the parts do not exist in isolation. There is an interrelationship of the parts. This demands looking at the parts in the context of the whole. There may be qualitative degeneration which cannot be set right by a quantitative approach, the approach of the dismantling of parts and reassembling them. The whole is not caught in the net of the parts. Even though the net may be very closely woven, the whole escapes from the holes of such an interwoven net. It is to this that Sir Arthur Eddington once referred, when he said that the scientist does not recognize the existence of that which has slipped out of his closely woven scientific net. And so the holistic approach is not the approach of totality. The whole is also not a many-sided view either. The many-sided view still is based on, quantitative perception. Just because one takes into account the many-sided view, one does not thereby come to the understanding of the whole. In the many-sided view, one is concerned with a statistical assessment. In such an assessment one arrives at an average. The average leads us to the understanding of the universal. We thereby cognize the mathematical reality but not the empirical reality. Dr. Carl Gustav Jung, the eminent psychologist, in his book, *The Undiscovered Self*, says :

> Scientific education in the main is based on statistical truths and abstract knowledge and therefore imparts an unrealistic, rational picture of the world in which the individual as a mere marginal phenomenon plays no role. The individual, however, as an irrational datum, is a true and authentic career of reality.

In all statistical averages one is concerned with a nonceptual reality and not an empirical one. Through statistical calculations one may come to the understanding of the universals but not the unique. The unique is matchless, one without a second. And in the stamp of life there is individuality or uniqueness. No two individuals are the same, no two events are the same. And, therefore, an approach of generlizations is bound to leave out something, and who knows that which has been left out may have crucial significance than that which comes within the framework of calculation? Each living human body has something unique which defies all processes of generalization.

It is not suggested that generalizations have no value. They are of great value for knowing the structure of things. They are of great help in understanding the parts and their structures. The human body is a machine, and yet it is not just a machine. The mechanical aspect of the human body needs a part-by-part approach just as one would do in examining the nature of a machine. Life does have its mechanical counterpart. But the difficulty arises when it is thought of as machine and nothing more. To understand the livingness of anything, one has to bring into one's understanding a new dimension, a dimension of the whole. It is in the perception of the whole that one is vouchsafed the understanding of the unique. There is an intimate relationship between the universal and the unique, between the part and the whole. It is like a relationship between the centre and the circle. The circle derives its meaning from the centre; in fact, the circle derives its very existence from the centre. And the centre is mysteriously present in every part of the circle. The very existence of the circle depends upon the centre. The centre and the circle are not opposites even as the whole and the parts are not. The whole is the intangible or, as David Bohm says, the implicate. The parts constitute the explicate. The parts have no meaning whatsoever unless they are seen in the background of the whole. The whole is in the parts but not of them. We have been discussing this question in relation to the problem of health or ill-health. One may ask : what is health? Surely, just the absence of illness is not health. Health is not the removal of the symptoms of ill-health. In fact, one may not have any symptom of illness, and yet one may not be healthy at all. Health is not something negative, it is supremely positive. Health is, indeed, wholeness. Anything that is fragmented and, therefore, torn away from the whole is ill. In subhuman kingdoms of nature, the parts torn from the whole are never to be seen. It is only with the arrival of man that such division between the parts and the whole is to be noticed. When the link between the parts and the whole is interrupted, the former is deprived of fresh and flowing energy. There is a blockage of energy, and this blockage is, indeed, the cause of all illness. Where there is a free and uninterrupted flow of energy, there is no trace of illness.

It is common experience that flowing water can never be dirty. It is the very flow that removes all elements of dirt. When the flow of water is blocked, stagnation arises. It is the stagnant water which is the begetter of all pollution and infection.

The germ theory of disease, which was the only prevalent theory some years ago in the field of medicine, has undergone much revision in recent time. The germ theory made the external or objective conditions the sole cause of disease. But now we find that the subjective factors have been indicated in the problem of disease. We are not going into the subtler aspects of the subjective factor here at this juncture of our discussion, but the one subjective factor recognized by all is the factor of body's immunity. It has been noted that some people are immediately prone to disease when they visit infected areas, but others are unaffected even while visiting the same infected areas. Why is this so? The main reason for such happenings is the immune system of the body. The human body has its own defence system which fights any incursion of foreign matter attacking the body from the outer polluted and infected surroundings. The human body has its own intelligence. Dr. Larry Dossey says in his book, *Space Time and Medicine* : 'Our own body contains the wisdom derived from countless challenges to its integrity. From the skin that covers us to the white blood cells that engulf invading micro-organisms, our body knows what to do.' Thus, the body knows what to do in given circumstances to maintain its condition unaffected by the outside invaders, the germs that arise from the polluted and infected areas. It is this intelligence of the body which maintains its immune system. It is most fascinating to study the mechanism of the immune system of the body by which it keeps itself unaffected by outer influences. But if this is so, why does the body become ill, why and how does its immune system break down ? A healthy body is very flexible in its functioning. It is able to adapt itself quickly to changing conditions. A body that is overprotected against changes of environment experiences a gradual breakdown of its immune system. A healthy body is one that is confident of facing outer environmental changes because of its capacity of quick adaptation. The body shows forth amazing capacity of adaptation due to its inherent intelligence. **Dr.** Larry Dossey says in the same book :

> Perhaps we should adopt a strategy wherein we try to behave not like an immovable Gibraltar but like bamboo, which in Oriental lore, bends with the wind instead of resisting it, and is thus preserved. Like a bridge that has no flexibility and can thus be shaken to pieces in a wind, our heroic and inflexible stance to resist being moved by disease, may doom us.

The body has innate flexibility by which it knows how to behave in a particular situation. This, indeed, is its innate intelligence. And it is this which keep intact its inborn immune system. When the immune system suffers from blockages, it becomes weak, and the body becomes an easy prey to infection. When the immune system becomes weak, the body experiences a loss of energy. In other words, the flow of energy is blocked, it is impeded, and that, indeed, is the cause of bodily illness. When the body has less and less energy at its disposal, it is unable to act with its innate intelligence; its natural defence mechanism gets shattered. In this problem of energy dissipation, mind-body interaction has to be taken into account.

In the whole problem of disease, neither body alone nor mind alone can be held responsible. Both together have to be taken into account. Sometimes there is a tendency to go to extremes, which is either treating the body alone without mind or treating the mind alone without taking into consideration the bodily factors. We suggest that there is a place for medicinal drugs but not the only place. Similarly, there is the place for the mental factors—but once again not the only place. Very often the medicinal drugs are forced to go beyond their limitations. The value of such drugs lies in the fact that they must keep the symptoms in a subdued state, not suppress them nor give them unbridled sway. The bodily symptoms have to be attended to, because they are the first manifestation of inner disorder. They must be kept in check so that they do not create further dissipation of bodily energy. Thus, there is a negative role which medicinal drugs can and must perform. But they by themselves cannot bring into operation the positive factors of health. The positive factors of health demand the removal of energy blockage wherever it may be. It is only the renewed flow of blocked energy that can produce positive factors of health.

It is very often seen that a person may not have any signs and symptoms of bodily ill-health. The investigations into the conditions of the different organs of the body may not show any condition of disorder, and these investigations may be through all the modern traditional and sophisticated instrumentation. And yet, in spite of all the negative reports, the body may not show forth conditions of health. For health requires a flow of vitality. A healthy body is a vital body, not merely a body free from the signs and symptoms of ill-health. It is this and certain other factors that create the vast problem of energy blockage.

In a human individual there are various centres of energy functioning. They are interrelated and cannot be considered in isolation. These centres are biological or physical, vitalistic, psychological and spiritual. It is only when there is a perfect synchronization in the functioning of these four centres that one can experience a state of complete health. These are the centres through which the human consciousness operates. And consciousness is whole, it cannot be compartmentalized. For the total well-being of a human individual the four-fold approach of consciousness is essential. There is a dissipation of energy at the level of the physical body, but there is also the dissipation of energy at other levels. And the dissipation is due primarily to the blockage of energy. It is, therefore, necessary to go into the whole question of energy blockage and energy dissipation at different levels before the problem of self-transformation can be successfully tackled.

3. The Nature of Time

IN THE whole subject of the depletion and dissipation of energy, the main factor to be considered is the flow of time. Man is for ever afraid of the flow of time, for it is believed that in the flow of time everything disappears, time brings everything to an end. In the *Bhagavad Gītā*, Lord Śrī Kṛṣṇa, while showing his universal form to his disciple, Arjuna, says: 'I am time devouring everything.' The movement of time is associated with death, for time brings everything to an end. Man has always been afraid of the flow of time because of its inescapable end in death. Modern science has denoted this movement of time and its effect by the term entropy. Its formulation comes in the Second Law of Thermodynamics. This law implies that the universe as a whole is moving steadily towards increasing disorder. As Peter Russell in his book, *The Awakening of Earth*, says: 'The Second Law of Thermodynamics states that in any energy interaction there is always a reduction in the amount of energy available to perform useful work.' This is the principle of entropy discernible in all fields of energy exchange. Everything is moving from order to disorder. This is the inexorable movement of time leading to death and destruction. This principle of entropy obviously indicates a steady movement leading to the loss of energy, thus breaking down the immune system of the organism. With the loss of energy, the in-built defence system of an organism collapses, thus reducing more and more its chances of survival. And we are told that this process of the depletion of energy is irreversible. This is also known as the arrow of time. The flow of time is irreversible. Although energy cannot be destroyed, yet this principle indicates that its transformation is such that it is no longer available to the organism for performance of any useful work.

15

The question of time demands a serious exploration. From the standpoint of science, time and space are not two distinct phenomena. Not only that. Time itself is relative. In other words, it depends upon the observer and his scale of observation. But, apart from this, there are two major aspects of time that need to be understood—it is time linear and non-linear. In the linear concept of time, there is a division with regard to the flow of time itself—it is a fragmentation of time into the past, the present and the future. This is time as an irreversible phenomenon. For it speaks of the past that has gone and the future that has not come. Its concept of the present is also made up of a little bit of the past and a little bit of the future. In this perception the present is a mere concept and not something which constitutes an empirical experience. It is just a dividing line between the past and the future having no intrinsic value. In this time evaluation the past is gone, never to return. It is this linear understanding of time which generates fear and fright about the passage of time. Time moves on and has never a moment when its movement stops. Time never stops, it moves on relentlessly towards its destination which is nothing but a total end. It is this which has generated in the minds and the hearts of the people a fear of death, and, therefore, of the relentless march of time. From the very beginning of the evolutionary history of humanity, man is seen fighting against the march of time. Is death the inevitable end of everything? If so, life has no meaning and purpose—this has been the thinking of men and women throughout the ages. But is there any other time than the irreversible movement indicated by the arrow of time? This movement signifies an ever-increasing entropy where energy is depleted and dissipated. Is not the principle of entropy an inexorable principle? Keeping aside for the time being the philosophical aspect of the phenomenon of time (we shall come to it later in this chapter), let us see whether science has anything else to offer except the irreversibility of time.

The movement of time in the linear sense, that is, along the arrow of time, is measured in terms of the loss of energy. It is measured in terms of entropy. This loss of energy signifies a process of irreversibility which means that the energy lost cannot be regained. But if science says that energy can neither be created nor destroyed, then what is meant by the irreversibility of energy? It is true that the sum total of energy in the universe is the same, that there can be neither increase nor dicrease in the store of energy. But then this does not rule out the possibility that a particular unit of life may just experience a non-availability of the energy that exists in the universe. And so for all practical purposes it experiences a depletion of energy, and it is said that this depletion cannot be made good. It is this energy loss and its irreversibility that is the cause of man's fear of the movement of time resulting in total annihilation or death. And man is for ever pitted against this passage of time. But since the movement of time cannot be stayed or controlled, man is intent upon packing the duration of time with as much of achievement and accumulation as possible. In other words, man is all the time in a hurry, so that, if he cannot stop the movement of time, he can at least achieve as much as possible during the availability of time duration. If the loss of energy cannot be made good, then let the available energy be put to highest use and as quickly as possible. In modern age, because of the quick tempo of life, there has come in the life of man a 'hurry sickness' as Dr. Larry Dossey says. In his book entitled *Space, Time and Medicine* he says:

Interestingly, the perceptions of passing time that we observe from our external clocks cause our internal clocks to run faster. . . . Our sense of urgency results in a speeding of some of our body's rythmical functions, such as the heart rate and respiratory rate. Exaggerated rises in the blood pressure may follow along with the increases in blood levels of specific hormones that are moved in the body's responses to stress. Thus our perceptions of speeding clocks and vanishing time cause our own biological clocks to speed . . . the end result is frequently some form of 'hurry sickness' expressed as heart disease, high blood pressure, or depression of our immune function, leading to an increased susceptibility to infection and cancer.

The linear perception of time brings into existence the speeding up of the internal [clock or the psychological time. A sense of hurry is created because of the running down of the clock. At the linear level of time-perception, the running down of the clock gives the feeling that something is lost which can never be recovered. The time gone is time lost for ever. And the running down of time is the relentless depletion of energy. With every advancing movement of time there is less and less energy left with which to tackle the problems of life. Time flies and with its flight we are left with less and less energy with which we meet the challenges of life. With the speeding up of the clock we tend to become older and older, because we associate the speeding of the clock with an ageing process which means more and more depletion of energy—the energy that is lost for ever and cannot be reclaimed. In a civilization like ours, built on advance technology and, therefore, of quick and rapid tempo, this experience of energy-loss is felt all the more. There is no wonder that modern man is terribly ill, for the lack of energy makes him more and more helpless to meet the impacts of life coming to him in quick succession.

But, then, is there a way out? Is not the movement of time linear and, therefore, irreversible?

Ilya Prigogine, the noted Belgian scientist, who was awarded Nobel Prize in 1977 for his discoveries, enunciates the theory of the reversible and the irreversible time. That time is reversible brings into focus the idea that time is not just linear, it is also non-linear. The linear time is obviously irreversible. In his epoch-making book, *Order Out of Chaos*, he develops the concept of reversible and irreversible time. It is said that while time is irreversible at the macroscopic level, it is reversible at the microscopic level. The understanding of this requires mathematical and technological insight, and so is beyond the ken of lay people. It is needless to say that the reversibility of time denotes that energy lost can be regained. It seems to be an anti-entropy movement. Energy gone is not gone for ever, it can be recovered. How is this possible and what is the explanation of this anti-entropy phenomenon? Peter Russell writes in his book, *The Awakening of the Earth* :

Life, however, would appear to contradict this trend. Living systems display a great deal of order. Every living being ... is a highly organised collection of energy and matter. And individual living systems not only retain a high degree of internal organisation, they build up this order as they grow and develop. Life appears to move towards increasing order rather than disorder. But according to the Second Law of Thermodynamics, a system such as your body should be gaining entropy. So does life somehow contravene a well-established and seemingly universal law of physics?

This is, indeed, a pertinent question. Is everything moving towards greater and greater disorder, gaining in entropy and ultimately ebbing out? Scientists tell us about the death of the universe because of the working of the principle of entropy. And yet life seems to be moving towards an order of greater and greater complexity. What is the explanation? Does life contravene the universal law of entropy enunciated by physics? Peter Russell states:

The answer is NO, and the reason is that the second law applies to closed systems—systems that are isolated from their environment such that there is no flow of matter or energy in or out of the system.

Living systems, however, are open systems, continually, exchanging matter and energy with their environment. Evidently in the functioning of the entropy principle there enters a change when one is concerned with the living system as against the non-living system. But is there such existence of the living and the non-living systems in the universe? It is true that life pervades everything, and so, strictly speaking, there is nothing inanimate. And yet there is a distinction between the living and the non-living systems. A living system has fundamentally three characteristics. Firstly, it displays a state of interrelatedness; in other words, it is not isolated. Secondly, this state of interrelatedness is active so that there is a constant interchange between the living system and its environment. It gives energy to the environment, and also receives in turn energy from the surroundings. Thirdly, the living system has a capacity for adjustment and adaptation. It is so flexible that it can show forth a quick adaptation to changing environment. As against this the non-living system is isolated, and, therefore, there is no interchange of energy. It obviously lacks a capacity for adaptation to changing situations. The living system is able to draw energy from life itself which is an inexhaustible store of energy, and so it does not function within the restrictive field of the Second Law of Thermodynamics. It does lose energy but is able to get back a fresh supply of energy from life itself. This is so because a living system is an open system, whereas the non-living system is a closed one. A closed system cannot draw energy from the environment. This is the fundamental difference between the open and the closed systems.

Physical science tells us that, in the operation of the principle of entropy, the organism reaches a point known as thermo-dynamic equilibrium. When this point is reached, there is no possibility of reversibility. Under this condition the unit of life has reached a condition of death because of the complete loss of energy. In the living system, however, there comes into being what is called by the scientist Prigogine a phenomenon entitled a Dissipative Structure. However, the emergence of this structure takes place before the thermodynamic equilibrium sets in. Needless to say, the emergence of such a structure is evident only in an open system. Thus, an openness of the system is an inescapable requirement for a reversal of the energy flow. Prof. Prigogine says that in a living system a gradual decrease of energy leads to a crisis or a critical point. This is called far-from-equilibrium state. At this point, a living system reveals an astonishing process of self-organization. One of the present-day scientists has written a book called *The Self-Organising Universe*.

Needless to say, such a process of self-organization can exist only in a living or an open system. But even here there is a pre-condition. Prigogine discusses this fascinating question in his book entitled *Order Out of Chaos*. What is this pre-condition? Dr. Larry Dossey speaks about this in his book, *Time, Space and Medicine.* It is this pre-condition which brings us to the fourth characteristic of a living or an open system. Dr. Larry Dossey says :

> . . . increasing complexity generates a need for increasing energy consumption from the environment which in turn gives rise to increasing fragility. But ironically it is this feature of the dissipative structure that is the key to its further evolution towards greater complexity. For if the internal perturbation is great enough, the system may undergo a sudden reorganisation, a kind shuffling, and escape to a higher order, organising in a new complex way. It is the quality of fragility, the capacity for being shaken up, that paradoxically is the key to growth. Structures that are insulated from disturbance are protected from change. They are stagnant and never evolve towards a more complex form . . . susceptibility is the catalyst for change.

This is, indeed, the fourth characteristic of a living or an open system. Curiously enough, it is fragility of the organism which enables it to enter a new order of living from the point of crisis. The critical point can serve as a catalyst ushering in a new and more complex state of living. As Dr. Larry Dossey says: 'Order could not arise without chaos.' But chaos arises when an organism is under the effect of entropy, and is in a state which is far from equilibrium. One can notice three states in nature's progression. This is equilibrium, near-equilibrium and far-from-equilibrium. When equilibrium comes, there is the end of the growing process. In conditions of near-equilibrium there may arise modifications or variations of structures. But it is only in the far-from-equilibrium state that mutations or fundamental transformations can arise. The far-from-equilibrium state is, indeed, a state of crisis, a state of highest perturbation. An organism which is insulated against this change must die—such is, indeed, the law of growth. Dr. Larry Dossey says :

> Recall, however, a central concept of dissipative structures : only through perturbation can the system escape to a higher

order of complexity. The key to growth is fragility. While
mild perturbances are damped within the system, major ones
are not; they have the possibility of stimulating a sudden
change toward a more complex system . . . evolution, says
dissipative structure theory, is impossible without fragility.
Perturbation and susceptibility to dissolution and death are
the prices to be paid for the potential for growth and complexity.

However our main concern in this book is not so much with
the growth and evolution at the physical and biological levels as
at the psychological level, for human evolution functions *par
excellence* at the psychological level. How do dissipative structures and fragility operate at the level of human evolution? Do
they contain any secret of transformation at the level of
humanity?

The principle of entropy functions as much at the physical
level as at the psychological level. With the passage of time
man, too, experiences a loss of energy, and the loss seems irreversible. Man is subject to the arrow of time as all units of
physical and biological nature. We saw earlier that Prigogine
speaks of the reversible and irreversible time. The first is per-
ceptible at the microscopic level, while the second is visible at
the macroscopic level. What about the human individual? Is the
loss of energy reversible? In other words, is time reversible at
the psychological level? Can the loss of energy be made good at
the human level? It is common place for us to say that everyone
is getting old, nobody is becoming younger. If that be the case,
reversibility has no relevance on man's field of existence. One
can say without any fear of contradiction that events are irreversible. A cup of hot coffee cools and never becomes hot again,
similarly an event happens and then it becomes a thing imbed-
ded in the past, never to be recovered. In other words, with
regard to events one has to accept the linear nature of time.
Here time flows in one direction, it moves along the path indicated by the arrow of time. It goes forward but never back-
wards. If this is, then it is surely irreversible. But has reversibility of time any relevance at the human level?

It has. While event is irreversible, the experience is undoubtedly reversible. One might say that while events belong to the macroscopic level, experience belongs to the microscopic level. The event is general but the experience is individual. We will not just at this stage go into the question as to how experience can become reversible. We shall do it later in the course of discussion. At this stage we want only to indicate that time can be experienced as reversible at the psychological level, and that this reversibility depends upon whether the human psychological system is open or closed. In a closed system there can be no experience of reversibility either of time or of energy. The open system is fragile and, as noted earlier, it is only through the condition of fragility that the unit of life can be initiated into a higher and a more complex order of existence. What is meant by fragility at the psychological level? The other two aspects in relation to the open system, namely, the capacity to adapt and the capacity of interchange of energy with the environment, would naturally follow from the conditions of openness. We will turn to the psychological aspects of growth under the impact of an open system in the subsequent chapters. Such discussion seems to be most essential to the process of self-transformation. We are told that fragility is the price that has to be paid for fundamental transformation. What are fragility and openness in the concept of psychological change? It is interesting to note what Lao Tze, the great Chinese philosopher, said about this many centuries ago. He says:

When the man is born, he is tender and weak;
    At death, he is hard and stiff.
When the things and plants are alive,
    They are soft and supple,
When they are dead they are brittle and dry.
Therefore hardness and stiffness
    Are the companions of death,
And softness and gentleness are the
    Companions of life.
Therefore when an army is headstrong,
    It will lose in battle.

When a tree is hard, it will be cut down.
The big and strong belong underneath.
The gentle and weak belong at the top.

Does the secret of self-transformation lie in the quality of soft-ness and gentleness? Is fragility the key to growth? In the chapters to follow we shall explore the implications of this strange theory of psychological mutations in the life of humanity, whether at the individual or at the collective level.

4. The Third Way

THE THEORY of dissipative structures propounded by Prof. Prigogine has great philosophical and psychological implications apart from its scientific overtones. The Second Law of Thermodynamics with its entropy principle has far-reaching meaning and significance. The Cartesian way has so conditioned our thinking that we see only the binary way of approaching everything. It is this binary way which has reached its summit in modern computer science, for all computers function on the binary principle. It is based on the dualism of either/or. It says that a solution to all problems can be found in the framework of opposites. A computer functions on the basis of the programme with which it has been fed. It can and does process the material with which it has been programmed. It does all the mathematical calculations —and that, too, extremely swiftly—but beyond the limits of programming it cannot go. It gives its answers on the binary principle. Our computers are digital in nature and so their feeding has to be done, one by one, in a sequential manner. It is said that the human brain is also a computer, but it is a computer with a difference and a distinction. Dr. Pfeiffer, an eminent brain scientist, in his book entitled the *Human Brain* says that while the brain is like a computer, there is no computer which is like the brain. This is because the human brain is not a digital computer but an analogue computer which receives its programme material, namely, sensations, all at once, not one by one as in the digital fashion. We talk today of the fifth generation computer which is described as artificial intelligence. However, artificial intelligence is not identical with creative intelligence. Mr. Hubert L. Dreyfus has written a book entitled *What Computers Cannot Do* with the subtitle *The Limits of Artificial Intelligence*. In it, the author

25

says that, while all types of formal feeding can be done with reference to a computer, it is not passible to feed a computer with common sense and insight. But man solves many problems with common sense, and common sense cannot be put on a programme chart. It cannot be worked out logically or mathematically. An intuitive flash cannot be worked out in advance. But without clear programming a digital and a binary computer cannot function.

Our thinking is by and large based on a binary principle. It knows an answer in terms of either/or. It cannot have any cognizance of the third way. But solutions to non-mathematical problems lie mostly along the third way. It is along the third way that one discovers the meaning of the mysterious statement 'more than both'. In the third way the two exist together, and yet the third way is not a compromise between the two. In the co-existence of the two there is something more than the sum total of the two. And it is this something more that the third way indicates. But to the mind of man the co-existence of the two is unthinkable. The binary process of thinking considers the co-existence of the two as meaningless. How can the opposites exist together? It is because of this that we have struggled for decades and centuries to find out what is true : determinism or freewill. We have all along considered that one of the two must be correct. For both cannot be regarded as correct. And yet Prigogine has shown in his theory, experimentally proved, that they both exist together. Alvin Toffler says in his introduction to Prigogine's book, *Order Out of Chaos*:

. . . according to the theory of change implied in the idea of dissipative structures, when fluctuations force an existing system into a far-from-equilibrium condition and threaten its structure, it approaches a critical moment or bifurcation point. At this point, it is inherently impossible to determine in advance the next state of the system. Chance nudges what remains of the system down a new path of development. And once that path is chosen, determinism takes over again until the next bifurcation point is reached.

Here we see chance and necessity not as irreconcilable opposites, but each playing its part as a partner in destiny.

Chance and necessity, freewill and determinism, existing together —this is the astonishing conclusion to which Progogine's theory leads us. We are forced to admit the existence of the third way. But curiously enough the third way cannot be defined, nor can it be determined in advance. It reveals itself. It cannot be worked out logically or mathematically in advance. It is not something with which a computer can be fed. And it alone shows the way out of chaos. It reveals itself at the bifurcation point. And as Prigogine says : '... we can never determine when the next bifurcation will arise.' The bifurcation point is something unpredictable. It can be known only when it comes. And so there seems to be in life a co-existence of the predictable and the unpredictable. The two opposites exist together, but it is only at the bifurcation or the critical point that the third way is found. The bifurcation point arrives only at the far-from-equilibrium condition where the dispersal of energy has taken place, and yet the thermodynamic equilibrium has not arrived. The unit of life is intensely unstable, going through intense perturbation, and yet the further degeneration of energy has been stopped. Such a critical state can arise only in a living or an open system and not in a closed one. Here one is reminded of the statement of another scientist, Le Comte du Nouy, who says in his book, *The Human Destiny*:

It is not the being best-adapted to his environment who contributes to evolution. He survives but his better adaptation eliminates him from the ascendent progression, and only contributes to increase the number of more or less stagnant species that people the earth. That smoothness of adaptation may be a hindrance to further advance is illustrated by the pre-Cambrian sand worms who achieved a very successful adaptation to their environment, and having no reason to transform themselves further, they subsisted almost without a change for hundreds of millions of years. One of these worms, however, continued to evolve because it was less adapted than the others and probably possessed a kind of instability which did not constitute an advantage at the time, but which was conducive to still greater changes and could be called creative instability. This worm, less perfect as a worm, may have been our ancestor.

We have seen that a closed system reaches a state of thermodynamic equilibrium which constitutes its end because of maximum entropy. It is only the living system that comes to a critical point at the state of bifurcation. But then the living system which is open has great flexibility because of which it can adjust and adapt to changing situations easily. But if it adapts, then it only survives for continuing a stagnant species. And so if it adapts, it dies, but then if it cannot adapt, then it is not a living or an open system in which case its death is inevitable. We seem to be in a paradoxical situation. We are on the horn of a dilemma, for neither adaptation nor non-adaptation solves the problem. What then is the way to resolve this paradox? When an organism has the capacity to adapt as living systems have and yet does not adapt, it comes, indeed, to the critical or bifurcation point. Not to have the capacity to adapt is the sign of a closed system, but to show forth adaptation is to come to a condition of equilibrium or death. To have the capacity and yet not to adapt is the sign of the crisis, a sign which denotes creative instability. This is the bifurcation point from where further movement cannot be predicted. It is here that the third way is revealed. We are, however, interested in discovering the third way at the psychological level, for the two-way approach of either/or is unable to solve psychological problems. We have seen that the third way reveals itself only at the bifurcation point—the point of crisis. But such a point is arrived at only when the system is open and not closed. Can one create conditions of openness at the psychological level, or has one to wait helplessly for it to arrive? The open system has a great capacity for adaptation and adjustment. But if it gets adapted, then the point of equilibrium is reached indicating a total end. If it has no capacity to adapt to newer and newer situations, then it denotes an existence, not of an open, but a closed system. Here we are faced with a situation which can be resolved only by the intelligence of the bambo. The bamboo neither resists nor does it succumb. It functions along the third way. The capacity to adapt to changed situations denotes openness of the system; but if it refrains from adaptation in spite of the capacity to adapt, then it discovers the third way. One of the former presidents of the Theosophical Society, Mr. C. Jinarajadasa, expressed this idea beautifully when he said: 'The thinking faculty tense and yet not thinking.' This is a critical point because of the capacity to think and yet not thinking. Why is there no thinking if the thinking faculty is able to function? An answer to this question cannot be given. It is something inexplicable, something that must remain unexplained to the field of the mind. And yet it is only when this point of the unexplained is reached that the third way is found.

This is a state which has been described as 'far-from-equilibrium'. In the open system there is a movement from the state of equilibrium of the closed system to a state known as near-equilibrium. If the mind acts from this point, then a variation, a modification can be created but not a mutation or a fundamental transformation. For this there has to be a further movement from 'near equilibrium' to 'far-from-equilibrium'. It is here that the dissipative structure comes into existence giving birth to the phenomenon of self-organization. In self-organization the unit of life enters into a new order of existence. But can this movement from near to far-from-equilibrium be brought about, and if so how? For it is at this critical or bifurcation point that the reversal of time or of energy flow can come into existence.

We have seen that the open system is flexible. In other words, it has the quality of catholicity and universality, for this is, indeed, the nature of openness. It is a quality of expansion. It has an element of confidence since it has the capacity of adaptation. In other words, it has a masculine quality of consciousness. This is the state where the thinking faculty is tense. There is an alertness which is indicative of openness. Without such alertness the system would be closed, having no adaptive capacity. But we have seen that the open system has also a quality of fragility. This is indicative of hesitancy. Needless to say, this is the feminine aspect of consciousness. A unit that is fragile is always hesitant. And so here we come across a paradoxical situation of confident and yet hesitant—the capacity to adapt and yet not adapting. There is tremendous tension which can be described as far-from-equilibrium. It is a turbulent state—a state where the critical or the bifurcating point has arrived. And it is at this point that the reversal of time and, therefore, of energy-flow comes into existence. The organism enters into an area of self-organization where, as it were, the reversal of entropy takes place. The organism is able to imbibe fresh energy from the environment, it is ready to start its new journey along the path of renewed organization. It is this fascinating implication to which one comes as one looks at the theory of dissipative structures of Prigogine when examined at the psychological level. It is certainly applicable to the biological aspect of life, but it is equally applicable, and with more revolutionary results, at the psychological level. In fact, herein lies the secret of self-transformation.

It is a known fact that energy can be released only when the two poles, the positive and the negative, meet. When an organism shows forth flexibility or catholicity and fragility or hesitancy, the meeting place of the masculine and the faminine has been reached where alone fresh energy can be released for the initiation of the self-organizing process. H.P. Blavatsky, the co-founder of the Theosophical Society, says in her priceless book, *The Voice of the Silence* : 'To live the mind must have breadth as well as depth.' The quality of breadth is the universal, the catholic quality which is masculine in its nature even as the quality of depth is indicative of feminine nature. Livingness is possible only when breadth and depth meet, when the masculine and the feminine co-exist. Strong and yet tender, confident and yet hesitant—this, indeed, is the nature of the living or the open system at the psychological level. Time is, indeed, irreversible, but it is also reversible. There is a running down of energy, but there is also a point from where fresh energy-flow comes into existence. From the critical point—and from there alone—a self-organizing process begins to function. In life there is both the process of reversibility and irreversibility. There is, indeed, the birth of order from chaos. The New Testament, the Christian scripture says : 'Blessed are the weak.' Blessed, indeed, are the fragile but their fragility is in the bosom of universality. This fragility is not born of weakness, for here we see confidence and hesitancy living together. Lao Tze, the great Chinese philosopher and mystic, says :

There is nothing weaker than water
But none is superior to it in overcoming the hard,
For which there is no substitute,
That weakness overcomes strength
And gentleness overcomes rigidity.

But the question is: how to arrive at this bifurcating point in life so that a reversal of the flow of energy takes place, so that one moves towards a fundamental transformation of life, both individual and collective? It is to this serious and deep inquiry that we must turn in the subsequent chapters.

5. *The Breakdown and the Breakthrough*

NATURE seems to be adopting a strange medium of communication, for it speaks in the language of paradoxes. Now in a paradox one sees the co-existence of seemingly opposite factors. They are like the koans of Zen Buddhism. Modern physics speaks of the wave and the particle, of freewill and determinism, of cause and effect and numerous such other factors which are contradictory in nature as existing together. Speaking about this strange factor, visible in modern physics, F. Capra in his book, *The Turning Point*, says :

> In the twentieth century, physicists faced for the first time a serious challenge to their ability to understand the universe. Every time they asked nature a question in an atomic experiment, nature answered with a paradox and the more they tried to clarify the situation the sharper the paradox became. In their struggle to grasp this new reality, scientists became painfully aware that their basic concepts, their language and their whole way of thinking were inadequate to describe atomic phenomena.

Werner Heisenberg is reported to have said : 'Can nature possibly be so absured as it seemed to us in these atomic experiments ?' The absurdity of nature seems to lie in the fact that nature uses the language of paradoxes to explain its activities. One such paradox is contained in the behaviour of entropy where at one place it presents the spectacle of a complete breakdown of a system, while at another place it shows the phenomenon of disorder breaking through into a more organized and complex order of organization. Both breakdown and breakthrough are presented by the functioning of the principle of entropy. There is no longer a question of either/or, but togetherness of both. Either entropy results in a breakdown or it results in a breakthrough, but how can it be an instrument for both ?

In the entropy phenomenon two conditions are discernible: (*i*) the condition of thermodynamic equilibrium; and (*ii*) the far-from-equilibrium condition. The former results in the breakdown of the organism and the latter presents the phenomenon of a breakthrough into a higher order or organization. How does this happen? Peter Russell in his book, *The Awakening Earth,* poses this question thus:

> ...even though living processes may not contradict the second law of thermodynamics, the question must be asked as to why an organism builds up and preserves a high degree of internal order. Why does a certain collection of atoms go against the trend of the rest of the Universe? Indeed, if the entire evolutionary process can be seen as one of increasing organisation, why does this happen within a Universe that is, as a whole, running down towards disorder?

This is a very pertinent question, for, if everything in the universe is running down, why should there be in this universal phenomenon a spectacle of breaking through into higher and more complex organization? Once again we are faced with the paradox of organization and disorganization within the same process of the functioning of the Second Law of Thermodynamics.

We have seen earlier that with reference to the entropy functioning there are two entirely opposite states: one of equilibrium and the other of far-from-equilibrium, the former resulting in total disorder and the latter resulting in a breakthrough into a higher and complex order. But there is also an in-between state which is known as near-equilibrium, that is, neither equilibrium nor disequilibrium but mid-point where, as we have noted earlier, variations or minor modifications in an organism can happen. This shows that there is a possibility of a slowing down of the movement of entropy. If there is a slowing down, then there can also be the possibility of accelerating the movement of entropy. How do these slowing down and accelerating processes function?

If the running down can be slowed, then how does this happen? For the near-equilibrium state must obviously be the result of the slowing down process. In this book we are primarily concerned with the entropy or the running down process at the psychological level. But before we go into the question of the two extreme manifestations of the entropy phenomenon, let us consider as to how the running down of energy at the psychological level happens, and what is the implication of such running down of energy? Needless to say, such running down of energy, both biological and psychological, is the cause of man's ill-health. In this running down there takes place an impairment of the inbuilt immune system of human organism. If this impairment can be slowed down, then the degenerating process can be halted. Regeneration will necessitate exploring the state of far-from-equilibrium condition where alone new order can come into existence. A further degeneration would obviously occur if the running down process resulted in a condition of total equilibrium. If near-equilibrium state could be maintained, then in that very act the degenerative process would be halted. It may be interesting to note that these three states—equilibrium, near-equilibrium and far-from equilibrium—are comparable to the three attributes or *gunas* about which Eastern psychology, particularly the psychology of the *Bhagavad Gītā* speaks. They are the *tamas, rajas* and *sattva*. The *tamas* is the state of inertia comparable to the state of thermodynamic equilibrium, *rajas* is the state of near-equilibrium, and *sattva*, too, is another aspect of the near-equilibrium. However, in the *Bhagavad Gītā*, Lord Śrī Kṛṣṇa asks his pupil, Arjuna, to rise above the three *gunas* or the attributes. It is the state beyond the three *gunas* which is comparable to the far-from-equilibrium state where alone mutations or fundamental transformations can take place. These four aspects become clearer when one examines the fourfold aspects of *karma* discussed in the *Bhagavad Gītā*. These are non-action, reaction, action and inaction. Non-action is obviously the state of intertia or *tamas*, the thermodynamic equilibrium. The reaction of the *Bhagavad Gītā* most assuredly denotes the state of *rajas* or the state of activity. The action of the *Gītā* refers to the state of *sattva*, very often translated as harmony. The condition of *sattva* has also to be transcended as indicated by the *Gītā*. Why should this be transcended ? It speaks of action, and surely action must denote the state of truly spiritual man. However, this state of *sattva* or action is only the opposite of *tamas*, action is most often the opposite of non-action. Thus it is a part of near-equilibrium condition. Action, so long as it is the opposite of reaction, belongs to the realm of the pairs of opposites. It is, indeed, the opposite end of *tamas* or inertia. Here the three-fold states denoted by the European philosopher, Hegel, explain the position in a clearer manner. He speaks of thesis, anti-thesis and synthesis, and he further states that synthesis in turn becomes the new thesis giving birth to its anti-thesis and so on. Here synthesis is only the opposite end of thesis. These three are somewhat similar to the *tamas*, *rajas* and *sattva* of the Eastern or more truly the Hindu psychology. And so *sattva* or action of the Hindu psychology is the opposite of non-action or *tamas*. Thus action and non-action are the opposites with the intervening factor of reaction or *rajas* of the Hindu psychology. Lord Kṛṣṇa asks his pupil to go beyond all the three—non-action, reaction and action, for they belong to the same category. In the terms used by Prigogine, reaction and action are near-equilibrium conditions even as non-action is a state of total or thermodynamic equilibrium signifying the condition of total entropy or the death of the unit of life. The *Bhagavad Gītā* speaks of the fourth state in the enumeration of the gospel of *karma* and that is inaction. It is inaction which is the far-from-equilibrium state. It is truly a crititical state where alone mutation or fundamental transformation is possible. The critical state of inaction does not last long, but during the split second that it lasts it gives birth to that which indicates the nature of the third way. The scientist, James Clark Maxwell, says :

...in the physical world, there are unpredictable moments when a small force may produce not a commensurate small

result but one of far greater magnitude. Every existence above
a certain rank has singular points—the higher the rank the
more of them. At these points influences whose physical
magnitude is too small to be taken account of by a definite
being may produce results of the greatest importance.

These singular points, indeed, are the critical points, they denote
the state of far-from-equilibrium. They are, indeed, the state of
inaction of the *Bhagavad Gītā*. This state of inaction is the
door to the third way. Commenting on the above idea of the
singular point of Maxwell, the great social philosopher, Lewis
Mumford of America, says :

At intervals, at critical moments, in crises, the human
personality may produce an effect out of all proportion to its
physical powers just as a tiny seed crystal dropped into a
saturate solution may cause the whole mass to assume a
similar crystalline form.

The far-from-equilibrium state is, indeed, a critical state in
which a qualitative revolution in the form of a mutation comes
into existence. This is, indeed, a state of inaction, not to be
mistaken for non-action. It is a condition of creative instability,
for it is far from a state of stability. For all practical purposes,
it is a fragile existence, totally insignificant and yet capable of
producing revolutionary effects. In Eastern philosophy, more
particularly the Indian philosophy, Yoga is considered a state of
equilibrium. But this state may well be described as a state far-
from-*tamas*—far from the state of thermodynamic equilibrium.
It is here that the state of disorder brings into existence a condition of higher order, the order of greater complexity. The
energy dispersal suddenly comes to a stop, and fresh energy is
available to the organism from environment itself. The energy
flow, and, therefore, the time flow has been reversed. And Yoga
has been defined by Sri Aurobindo as reversal of consciousness.
Jesus said in the Sermon on the Mount that it is 'only as you
become like little children can you enter the Kingdom of God'.
H. P. Blavatsky says in her book, *Voice of the Silence*, that 'the

rose must become the bud'. All these statements denote a process of reversal. And this is a precondition for far-from-equilibrium state, the state of the bifurcation point or the state of the singular point. But before one comes to the far-from-equilibrium state in terms of psychological process, one must look at the near-equilibrium point where the flow of energy is slowed down, not halted, but slowed down. This means the slowing down of the dispersal of energy. And this has to be considered in the context of the living or the open system. As we have stated, we must consider this at the psychological level, for that is our main sphere of interest.

It is needless to say that in the process of living, energy is bound to be expended. Without the use of energy one cannot live. But it is one thing to use energy, and it is quite different to dissipate energy. If dissipation could be halted, then it is possible to come to the condition known as near-equilibrium. If this dissipation is not halted, then the organism will speedily move towards a condition of thermodynamic equilibrium which means total annihilation of the state of death so far as the organism is concerned.

Now, coming to this near-equilibrium condition has much to do with the problem of ill-health. One must first deal with the problem of ill-health before one comes to the positive experience of health. The positive experience of health demands coming to the far-from-equilibrium state. But before that experience of positive health, one must deal with the problem of ill-health. This is what is indicated by the slowing down of the downward flow of energy. This is the symptomatic approach to the problem of ill-health. This must be the starting point. It may be stated again that the body and the mind are in a state of constant interrelationship. And so the symptomatic approach has to be with regard to the body and the mind together. If one were to move along without staying at the state of near-equilibrium, then it is not the far-from-equilibrium state which will be experienced; it will be the state of total equilibrium, the state of total extinction. This is what very often happens in man's psychological journey when at the instance of somebody the person throws up all the props that had sustained him so far. Thereby he does not come to a critical point, the state of vulnerability, but rather to a state of utter confusion leading not to a new order but rather to a condition of unmitigated darkness, a state of unbroken inertia. That is why a stop-over at the near-equilibrium state is essential before one comes to the state of positive health, of wholeness. But how?

This requires an understanding of the process of ill-health— of how it proceeds, how it gathers intensity—ill-health of the body and the mind.

In the near-equilibrium state there are visible the signs and symptoms of disorder, of a bodily and mental malaise, of discomfort, of effects of maladjustment. Either the symptoms are sought to be suppressed or they are allowed to grow unchecked. Both these approaches produce the same result which is the running down of the organism, its energy totally dissipated; in one case the dissipation is due to resistence, in the other case it is due to indulgence. Either of these cannot solve the problem; in fact, both lead to the state of *tamas* or the thermodynamic equilibrium, neither the suppression nor the proliferation of symptoms. Then what? Is there a third way of dealing with the problem of ill-health?

There is an immune system both of the body and of the mind. The third way is to see that the immune system is not weakened. This is the work that can be done at near-equilibrium state. The strengthening of the immune system happens at the critical point of far-from-equilibrium state. But not to weaken the immune system or to temporarily halt the flow of energy dispersal—the halting of the further running down of the system—both of the body and the mind—can happen at the near-equilibrium state. This must be the first consideration in dealing with the problem of ill-health.

Every living organism has its immune system which contains the strength and the vitality of that organism. It contains its inherent intelligence to look after itself. The first consideration in dealing with the problem of ill-health must always be to see that the functioning of this innate intelligence of the organism is not impaired. So far as the body is concerned, this requires taking a proper note of one's habits with regard to food, exercise as well as rest. Any habit which becomes entrenched and, therefore, constitutes a factor of rigidity serves as a blockage for the smooth flow of energy. It is, therefore, necessary from time to time to bring about changes in the pattern of one's living. Of course, such changes cannot be at the cost of general well-being of the body. And so, within the general laws of health, it is necessary to bring about changes in one's pattern of living at the physical level. This will keep up the livingness of the body system. The immune system of the body and the mind constitutes their capacity for endurance and containment. A healthy body and a healthy mind can endure numerous impacts that come from the environment. This endurance must be preserved. This denotes one's confidence in the functioning of the body and the mind. If the confidence is lost, then the body and the mind do not and cannot function effectively. One has to find out the endurance limits. These limits should not be stretched too far, but they must be extended a little from time to time. An organism that is too protected tends to be demoralized. It loses confidence in itself. Of course, there can be no hard and fast rules about this. One has to find out by personal experience and experimentation. The organism must not be smothered by too much protection. If this rule is observed, then the endurance capacity of the organism tends to increase. Once again one has to follow the middle path of neither mortification nor indulgence. Anything that weakens or depresses the endurance capacity can never be conducive to health maintenance of the body or the mind. It is here that the question of bodily medication needs to be examined. The purpose of medication must be neither to suppress the symptoms nor to induce their proliferation. If medication seeks to take over the legitimate functions of the body, then it cannot be beneficial. Most often strong medication tends to depress the immune system of the body. The so-called wonder drugs are most often than not factors that depress the immune or the endurance system of the body. Very often they eliminate the symptoms by suppressing them and in this operation create what are known as 'side effects'; and these side effects are more dangerous than the principal illness itself. The symptoms are suppressed, but bodily health is not restored.

While medication sometimes may become necessary, it must be to the end of strengthening the immune and the endurance system of the body. The purpose of medication must not cross this barrier. Help nature and work on with her is the soundest law to follow. The process of medication must not subvert the innate functioning of body's immune system. Very often over-medication and unwise medication hasten the process of entropy leading the body to a state of inertia or thermodynamic equilibrium. Medication and other such devices must at best maintain the near-equilibrium state and not push the organism to the condition of total equilibrium of complete inertia, which is only another name for the death of the system.

In dealing with all problems of ill-health, the condition of the mind has to be taken into account. Mind, too, has its immune system, and this again is its endurance capacity or more particularly its containment ability. Just as over and unwise medication prevents the body to regain its state of health, the condition of the mind, too, may move towards greater and greater entropy, towards a running down state with ever-increasing loss of energy. This happens when the mind is subjected to quick and instant reactions. In such reactions of the mind, its energy gets lost and with it there is lost its flexibility and its pliability due to the energy loss. It tends to become irritable, unable to contain the impacts and the impulses of life. The mind that has a capacity to 'contain' denotes a condition of health and vitality. The mind that immediately reacts is a shallow mind. Its reaction is its defence mechanism, and the mind that needs to put up defence mechanism has no confidence in its own innate capacity to meet the situation of life. It has less and less confidence for its survival, and this very fear impairs its immune system. Very often a person thinks that if he does not react immediately, his 'image' will be shattered and other people will think that he is a weakling, unable to stand up against the outer impact. But the fact of the matter is that immediate reaction is a sign of weakness; that he who can contain the impact, whatever its nature may be, is truly a strong person, rooted in a deep confidence so that he need not be afraid of being uprooted by impacts and incursions emanating from the outer environment.

We have seen earlier that wisdom lies along the third way which speaks of the coexistence of confidence and hesitancy. The sense of confidence will move towards arrogance and over-confidence when hesitancy is not there; similarly, hesitancy will move towards weakness and spinelessness when confidence does not coexist with it. As we have seen the third way denotes a state of far-from-equilibrium condition. It is a critical point or the bifurcation point. But one can come to it only if the innate immune system of an organism is not weakened either by suppression or proliferation. The body and the mind must maintain their immune or endurance capacity, for thus alone it will be able to come to a point of creative instability where a mutation or a new order can come into existence. The critical state is the state of fragility but it is not a state of weakness. There is the coexistence of fragility and agility—agile and yet fragile that is the nature of the critical state. It is the critical state which opens the door to the third way.

The American anthropologist, Casteneda, in his numerous books shares with the world the teachings which he has received from his American Indian teacher, Don Juan. At one place his teacher told him : 'Twilight is the door to the Unknown.' The twilight is the threshold that leads to the third way, for in the twilight there is the coexistence of the two—the day and the night. The twilight is the critical point, the bifurcation point. It is the point of creative instability.

But then the question is : how to come to this experience of the twilight in terms of human consciousness?

6. The Spiral Movement

THE main theme of this book as indicated in the very title is to seek out the secret of self-transformation. In the ultimate analysis all real transformations have to be self-initiated. Any transformation that has its initiating point outside is very superficial, it is only a change of behaviour pattern. We have seen so far in our discussion that, at the biological level, living system comes to a critical point where takes place the awakening of the process of self-organization. From that point the biological living organism initiates a new and a more complex order of organization. This seems to be the way of nature with regard to living systems at the biological level or even at the level of mineral life as evidenced in the behaviour of certain crystalline organizations. But with the arrival of man a new factor comes into operation, and that is the human mind. Man is not entirely at the mercy of nature, although he cannot work at cross-purposes so far as nature is concerned. If the mind of man functions with the propensities of nature, then it is possible for him to accelerate the movement of the living stream. In other words, at the psychological level there is a possibility of speeding up the process of self-organization. In fact, that which hastens can also retard. It all depends as to whether the mind of man works with nature or works against it. If mind can help nature, then nature's movements can be speeded up, otherwise there comes into existence a process of retardation. Nature allows man to take liberty with her up to a certain point; after that, it recoils. And such recoiling can be seen today when medication crosses its legitimate limits. Not merely in the sphere of health, but even in other spheres one can see the recoiling by nature due to man's efforts of moving in the direction of subverting nature or

42

attempting to replace nature. Evolutionary process can be speeded up, and that, indeed, is the purpose and technique of Yoga.

It has to be remembered that it is the living system alone that can come to the breakthrough point of a new order. This happens through the process of self-organization that comes into operation when the living and the open system arrives at a critical point. It is at this critical point that there is a search for the meeting point between stillness and motion, between time arrested and time passing. Among the Hindu sculptures the Dancing Śiva symbolizes this meeting place of stillness and motion. It is this which is the characteristic of a living system coming to the critical point as it opens the door to a new order. Under certain conditions entropy itself becomes the progenitor of order. But can this critical point be predicted? Prigogine says that one does not know when the next bifurcation point will arrive. In other words, it is an unpredictable event; it represents randomness or chance in the evolutionary scheme. If that be the case, then how can there be a speeding up or an acceleration of the self-organization process? Surely, one cannot bring the critical point at one's will. It looks as if one must resign oneself to the vagaries of nature. This probably is so in the sphere of biological life. But there seems to be a change when one arrives at the psychological field of growth and development. This is because of the human mind which has within it the power to speed up nature's movement. The junction between stillness and motion is, an intangible point, and so it comes only when it will. The unpredictable, the random, is outside the movement of predictability. And yet it is possible to prepare an organism to reach the threshold point. From the point of the threshold no further movement can be organized. It is really a point of stillness, and there, and only there, the arrival of a new movement—of a new order—can take place. In an open system the disorder itself, the entropy itself, becomes the progenitor of order. Surely, the new order cannot be predicted, nor can there be a speeding up of the arrival of such an event. But an organism can open itself out of newer and newer fluctuations or perturbations so that it goes nearer and nearer to the point of vulnerability. When all the defences of the organism get removed, it becomes completely defenceless or totally vulnerable. And the unpredictable can arrive only in the area of total vulnerability. The movement towards vulnerability can be speeded up, but only in a living or an open system. The state of vulnerability is, indeed, the condition of fragility, but the way to the state of fragility is through the gateway of agility. The agile is the quick moving, it is far from the state of inertia. The experience of stillness comes not to the dull mind but only to the agile or the quick moving mind. And the quick movement can be made quicker, for this is within the purview of the human mind. It is only such a mind that can come to the critical point. The dull mind never knows the arrival of the point of bifurcation. It is only in the waking state that the awareness of the point of bifurcation comes. This is awareness with choice. An agile mind knows what are the options before it, what are the factors of choice in front of it. The human mind can quicken its pace towards this point. When all the choices and their implications are seen, then does the mind come to a point of no further choice. And this, indeed, is the critical point—a point leading nowhere. This is, indeed, the point of utter chaos where no further movement is discernible. It was the great European philosopher, Nietzsche, who said; 'One must still have chaos in one to give birth to a dancing star.' The agile mind alone can know fragility. It is at the point of utmost fragility that the junction of stillness and movement is reached. It is here that the reversible and the irreversible meet.

In our discussion of the nature of time we saw that modern physics speaks about the reversible and the irreversible time. It appears that time is both reversible and irreversible. Science tells us that at macroscopic level time is irreversible, but at the microcosmic level it is reversible. We are not going into the mathematical and technical subtleties of this question. But we saw that, at the psychological level too, the reversibility and irreversibility of time can be noted and experienced. We said that an event is irreversible, but an experience is reversible. The event is general or one might say macroscopic. But an experience is personal or particular and hence microscopic. And, indeed, personal aspect of an experience can be seen as reversible. The linear time is irreversible, the past as an event is gone and cannot be brought back. The hot cup of coffee in terms of time becomes cold, and it cannot become hot once again by itself. The event is gone belonging as it does to the general or the macroscopic world. And yet the experience of an event can be revived or can be known as reversible. Time, indeed, is irreversible as well as reversible. And the flow of time is the flow of energy. Thus, it is possible to witness a reversible process in the flow of energy. The energy lost can be regained. But how? This is possible only at the critical point. And the conditions necessary for the arrival of the critical point can be advanced by the activities of the human mind. What nature does after a long duration of time can be expedited by the processes of mind at the psychological level.

While discussing the nature of time we said that the common view of time is that it is linear in its flow. This is what is called the arrow of time. According to this view, time is irreversible. In terms of Prigogine's view, the reversibility and irreversibility are associated with the predictable and the unpredictable phenomena of life. That which is unpredictable is irreversible. That which belongs to randomness or chance is obviously unpredictable. The reversible is repeatable. But this repeatable concept requires consideration of time as cyclic.

Is time linear or is it non-linear? Or is time both linear as well as non-linear? We have noted the paradoxes of nature to which physics draws our attention where two seemingly opposite things exist together. Are we faced with a similar paradox in the flow of time? The flow of time seems to vary in differing systems. In the mechanistic or close system time is most assuredly linear. It strictly follows the path indicated by the arrow of time. Here the flow of time presents the phenomenon of a running down process. At the mechanistic level, the universe is seen as a running down phenomenon where the entropy increases until the point comes where total equilibrium or *tamas* is reached. This is the point of extinction so far as the mechanistic unit is concerned. The clock runs down and it cannot wind itself so as to function. All mechanistic systems, being closed systems, have no self-organizing processes. This is the linear flow of time or energy.

But when we come to biological or living system we witness

a different flow of time. The biological systems are open systems where the interchange of energy takes place between the organism and the environment. Here we see not the linear but a cyclic flow of time. This can be seen in the changing colours on the leaves of trees during autumn and spring. As the English poet, Shelley, says: 'If winter comes, can spring be far behinds?' Autumn and winter and spring seem to show forth the interesting phenomenon of the cycle of seasons. The spring goes but comes back again, and this circle goes on in an unending manner. The same phenomenon of the cyclic flow of time is perceivable in the behaviour of birds and animals. The migrating birds fly thousands of miles on the onset of winter and again return to their original habitat when the fury of the season is lessened. This goes on year after year. Animals, too, have their seasonal behaviour. And so, at the biological level, time moves not in a linear fashion but in a cyclic manner. There is the cycle of events, a recurring phenomenon. There is seen in the flow of time a factor of reversibility. Time is irreversible at the machanistic level, but it is reversible at the biological level.

But there is still another category of time, and that is psychological. At the psychological or human level, the flow of time receives still another dimension, and that is psychological. At this psychological level, time is not only cyclic, it is also spiral. In the cyclic nature of time, there is a recurrence of events, but this is at the same point. In the spiral movement, however, the recurrence is not at the same point but at a little higher level. Every spiral returns to its earlier point but at a little higher level. This is the flow of time at the human or psychological level. Thus, there are three categories of time—mechanistic, cyclic and spiral. The spiral movement is also cyclic but with a difference. In the spiral phenomenon there is the coexistence of the horizontal and the vertical. The recurrence is not exactly at the same point but vertically a little higher. We saw earlier that, while events may disappear in the linear movement of past, present and future, the experience can be recovered. We saw that while the event is general, comparable to the macroscopic aspect, the experience is individual or microscopic. We said that while the event is not reversible, the experience can be. But experience does not exist by itself; it arises out of the event. And so, if the event does not recur, how can there be the recurrence of the experience? But, at the psychological level while the recurrence of event may not take place, the human mind has the capacity to recreate the event. And the recreation is tantamount to the recurrence of the event. It is only when the event is recreated that the experience can be regained. And the regaining of the experience is, indeed, regaining of energy. Thus, the energy that is lost can be regained through the recreation of the event at the psychological or human level. The immunity of the body and the mind which gets lost in the movement of time can be regained because of the recreation of the event. And the recreation of the event is the reversal of time. Time moves forward, but it also moves backward. This recreation and the reversal arising therefrom is possible only at the psychological level where time unveils a movement which is not only cyclic but spiral as well. The event and the experience are a joint phenomenon; they cannot be separated. If experience denotes the energy phenomenon, then surely there must take place the event phenomenon too. We shall discuss in great detail this recreational capacity visible at the psychological level in the subsequent chapters, and with that we shall see how energy lost can be regained.

It has, however, to be understood that the renewal of energy denotes the birth of the self-organizing phenomenon. At the mechanistic level, there is no self-organizing activity, because here we are dealing with a closed system. At the biological level, we come to a living or an open system where from the point of crisis there emerges a new order. But here the arrival of the critical point is entirely in the hands of nature—there is no possibility of the speeding up of the process. At the psychological level, too, the self-organizing movement can begin only from the point of crisis. Here, too, the critical or the bifurcation point must be reached. However, at the psychological level, the movement towards the critical point can be speeded up. Nature can be induced to move faster, so that the bifurcation point is reached earlier. This is really the recreation possibility of the event. It is through recreation that the critical point can be reached. Thus, the reversal of time at the psychological level is possible only through the recreative activity of the human mind. The recreative power at the psychological level is the power of imaginative visualization of the human mind. The bifurcation point is the point of fragility, for the mind does not know which way to go. It is fragile but not fickle. It is with the tremendous agility of the mind that it comes to the fragile moment of not knowing which way to take from the junction of bifurcation.

The agile mind is, indeed, an intelligent mind. But what constitutes the intelligence of the mind? Surely the mind that knows what its possibilities are and is also aware of its limitations is, indeed, an intelligent mind. Now it is not necessary that a person should physically go through all the experiences before becoming aware of the possibilities and the limitations of the human mind. This awareness can come, and come most effectively, through a vicarious process. One can vicariously move nearer and nearer to the bifurcation point. The bifurcation point brings one face to face with the unknown. At that point the mind of man proclaims that 'it does not know where to go'. This is the moment of highest intelligence. One comes to this point by and after actually examining all options and alternatives to life's situations. But then this process is time-consuming. It may take years and years to come to that point, and even then one may not come to it at all. However, it is possible to come to this point vicariously, that is, by the use of imaginative visualization. By this process not only can the past be recovered but the future, too, can be expedited. It is by imaginative visualization that one can operate, and operate successfully, on the flow of time at the psychological level.

Generally, time is classified as factual and personal. Factual time is, indeed, the biological time. This is time according to the movement of the biological clock. The flow of the mechanistic time is measured in terms of the movement of the man-made clock. The clock time is not the factual time. In fact, it is relative time, for it differs from area to area. Besides, clock time can be advanced or put back according to the exigencies of man. The clock time is based on social convenience. The real factual time is the biological time, for it depends upon the movement of the vital force or energy. It is the rate at which nature functions.

It is the third category of time, neither the clock time nor the biological time, but the personal time that constitutes man's acute problem. It is not the factual time but the fictitious time which is brought into existence by the mind of man. Man feels constrained by the movement of this time which has been created by himself. He is the creator of personal time, and feels eternally enchained by it. He goes hither and thither wanting to be free from its bondage. He creates it and feels constrained by it. But the question is: what is personal time, and how does it operate? It is a time superimposed by the mind of man on the normal passage of biological time. It is a superimposition of fiction over fact. How does this happen and why does man create this fictitious time?

Man's life is filled with events, some pleasant and some painful. There may be events that are neutral, but then such neutral events do not create any problem at all. It does not matter whether they come or they do not come, whether they endure or they do not endure. It is the pleasant or the painful events that pose problems to man, very often insurmountable problems. But is any event pleasant or painful by itself? Events are neither pleasant nor painful by themselves. It is man who makes it so. How does this happen? All events come and go, they follow the trend of the biological movement. They are the products of the passage of the factual time. An event comes in time duration and goes in the same duration of factual or biological time. It is in their passage that the mind of man seeks to intervene. This is done by wanting the event to continue or wanting the event to end immediately. He wants the events that awoke pleasant sensations from within him to continue and those that evoke painful sensations to cease to continue. But the events come and go in the natural flow of time. When an event ends physically but continues within the mind of man, a gap is created between what has happened physically and not inwardly. It is in this gap that personal time comes into existence. There is a curious phenomenon of the physical event and personal event. The first is factual but the latter is fictitious. When the physical and the personal events do not synchronize, time and its movement create enormous problem. It is not a real problem, it is entirely fictitious, and is created by mind of man. If the physical and the personal events could synchronize, then there would be no problem at all. In fact, one comes to the experience of positive health only when there is synchronization at all levels, including the personal and the psychological. After all time is one but its measurement differs from the mechanical to the biological and from there to the psychological levels. At the psychological level, the difficulties arise when the personal superimposition or projection comes into operation. Bertrand Russell says that we all live in our own private worlds. The world is the same but we project personal factors upon it and create a personal world with its own time duration. Then the factual time looks too long or too short, according to the personal mood of thinking and experiencing. While time at the mechanical level cannot be altered because of its close system, the time duration can be hastened or retarded where living or open systems operate. Thus, at the biological level, the hastening of time is possible, and this is what science has been doing all the time by crossbreeding and crosspolination in the animal and plant realms. New species in the animal and the vegetable world are being constantly created by scientific processes, thus hastening the process of nature at the biological level. Similarly, this hastening process can be done, and is being done, at the psychological level too. This is what the Yoga strives to do under a variety of approaches. But this is possible only where the two categories of time completely synchronize. When this is done, the transformation of the human individual is brought about, not at the biological but at the psychological level. In fact, at the human level there is a shift in the evolutionary process from biological to psychological. Humanity here rises to a new spiral in its evolutionary journey.

The hastening of the time duration is possible only in living or open systems. This requires the reaching of the critical point where the process of self-organization comes into existence The self-organization process can be hastened or delayed at the psychological level depending upon the synchronization or non-synchronization. If synchronization is the key to healthy growth, then the question arises as to how it can be brought about. It is only when the factual and the personal processes function at cross-purposes that energy gets depleted leading to the end of the organism. When the personal movement of time is not super-imposed on the factual realm, the critical point is reached quickly giving birth to the self-organizing process leading up to a new order of existence.

But how is this synchronization to happen? How can the personal and the factual meet at the same point, at the same time and with the same intensity? Such meeting alone is true synchronization. The only instrument which man poses for the synchronization of the personal and the factual is the technique of imaginative visualization. What is it and how does it function—into these questions we must go as we proceed with our discussions in the next chapter.

7. The Field of Memory

TIME is, indeed, a great mystery, for the flow of time is one thing and the sense of time is something else. There is, as we have seen, the social or the clock time, there is again the biological time which is identical with the flow of life. But there is also psychological, or more truly, the personal time. It is this flow of time which constitutes a major problem in the life of a human being. When we describe one category of time as psychological what we really mean is the flow of time with reference to psychological events. It is with reference to the flow of time in regard to psychological events or happenings that personal time comes into existence. The events of a psychological nature also happen at the objective level. The objective is not necessarily material or physical. It can be, and, often is non-material and, therefore, non-physical. The objective happenings are, thus, of a twofold nature—material and non-material. Into all non-material happenings man does not always project a personal factor. But it is also true that into some material happenings man does project personal factors. In other words, personal factors are projected on to all happenings in which man's psychological involvement seems to operate. This can be with reference to objects or persons or even ideas. It is this psychological involvement which brings personal time into existence.

When there is a personal involvement in anything, whether objects, persons or ideas, one does see the operation of personal time. In this context even physical happenings become psychological. It would be more appropriate to call this the flow of personal time. The question is: from where do the personal projections come, and how do they come?

This question involves exploring the vast and the complex field of memory. Memory is, indeed, not only very complex, it is also extremely mysterious. Modern psychology is trying to unravel the mystery of memory. It was thought that memory resides in certain specific areas of the brain. But, with the holistic approach discernible in all scientific thinking, the question of memory centres is also undergoing change. It is presumed that the whole of the brain is involved in memory storage. But memory is not just confined to the brain, although there is an aspect of memory which can be called brain memory. There is memory at the subhuman levels too. Psychometry, a branch of parapsychology, refers to memory stored by so-called inanimate objects. Those who have psychic or paranormal powers can psychometrize these objects, and can find. out whatever the objects have stored by way of memory. This memory record is absolutely correct, because no psychological or subjective factors have been projected. But this memory is not available to all, because it is only those who possess paranormal faculties alone can unravel the mystery stored in an inanimate object. But apart from this grade of memory there are other grades and levels of memory too. There is the chronological memory just as there is psychological memory which essentially is a personal memory. There is an associative memory just as there is a retentive memory. There is also the visualized memory which is dependent upon man's imaginative faculties. Thus memory is spread over a wide field. It is at the conscious level as also at the subconscious level. There is also the social or the racial memory about which the psychologist, Carl Jung, spoke. It is the memory of the unconscious. Although the field of memory is vast, in the present book we are concerned with the psychological or personal memory. This includes the visualized memory too, for it is this which enables the human individual to bring within his knowledge the spiral nature of one's experience. As we have seen earlier, while the event is irreversible, the experience belongs to the category of reversibility.

The question is: from where does psychological or personal memory arise? We know that the chronological memory has its roots in the chronology of events. But which is the ground in which personal memory resides? From this arises another question: who sustains this personal memory? Patañjali defines memory in his Yoga Aphorisms by saying that the memory is the effort of the human mind not to allow the experienced events to be stolen away. It is an effort of the human mind to hold on to the events that have ended chronologically. In other words, from the non-synchronization of the chronological event and the psychological event comes into existence what we have called the psychological or the personal memory. The event is over chronologically, but the mind still holds on to the event as if it is still happening. This is, indeed, the birthplace of personal memory. At the chronological level it has no validity. To give validity to the chronologically non-valid event is the *modus operandi* of personal or psychological memory. When an event leaves behind a hang-over, the psychological or personal memory is born. A state of hang-over indicates a condition of incomplete experience. In fact, an incomplete experience is the ground in which personal memory takes its root. An incomplete experience denotes a non-synchronization of the event and the experience. The event has been completed, but the experience thereof remains incomplete. It is the incomplete experience which brings into existence psychological or personal time. It creates a psychological future in which to complete the incomplete experience. The eminent thinker of our age, J. Krishnamurti, used to say again and again that there is no psychological future. It is something fictitious which the mind of man has created. What exists psychologically is the present—what the philosophers have called the eternal now. Everything exists only in the now. But when that which has happened in the now is incompletely experienced, then the so-called future comes into being. The past and the future have certainly a meaning in the chronological sense, but psychologically they do not exist. But the incomplete experience wants a future in which completeness of an experience can be known. But for the completion of this incomplete experience one demands a continuity of the event. Since an experience has come in the context of the event, it is quite natural that a desire for the continuity of the event, is demanded. Thus is man lost in the frustrating process of demanding the continuance of an event. However, life is in a state of eternal flux, nothing stands still, not even for two minutes. When the event does not stand still man resents and protests against the cruel way of fate. Thus do time and its passage become a never-ending problem for man. It is needless to say that the clock time is no problem at all, for it can be advanced or put back according to social needs. The clock time is the time created by society for its needs and requirements. Similarly, biological time is a fact of nature against which no will of man can prevail. It is the flux of life itself. It is the nature of life. It is only psychological or personal time that poses a problem. It becomes a problem, for man wants to control the movement of biological time in terms of the personal time. Man wants life to halt in pursuance of his requirements as specified by the movement of personal time. He wants the movement of the event to slow down so as to give him time to complete that which has remained incomplete. When this does not happen, man becomes prematurely old. If he accepts the onset of age without becoming old, he would be free from the impossible demands of the psychological or personal memory.

But then what about the incomplete experiences? Without extension of time-duration how can the incomplete experience be completed? And without such completion how can man be free from the pulls of the events that have gone? Time must stop for a while if man is to know satisfaction and fulfilment. And if time does not stop, then how can the incomplete experiences ever be completed?

But one may put a counter-question: can an experience be ever completed in time? One has to inquire as to what the nature of psychological time is. From where does it emerge? Surely, what we have called the personal or the psychological time exists only in the movement of thought. The movement of the mind is the movement of thought, and it is this movement which brings into existence personal time. Now mind can function only by the movement of thought. And so the personal or the psychological time is nourished and maintained by the movement of thought. In fact, the movement of thought is synonymous with the movement of personal time. Now a completion of experience denotes a state of discontinuity. Can an experience be ever completed in the continuity of personal time? The obvious conclusion is that, for the completion of an experience, it is not the continuity of time but the cessation of time that is necessary. In fact, the cessation of thought is the completion of experience. It needs not time and more time but a cessation of time. It is the rent in the veil of personal time that indicates the completion of an experience.

We have seen that psychological memory is the creator of personal time. Now, with the holistic approach becoming more and more acceptable in all fields of life, memory, too, has to be understood in a holistic approach. Dr. Roger Jones in his very fascinating book, *Physics as Metaphor*, says: 'Memory is everywhere, not spread out in the brain.' It is not the left or the right hemisphere which is the repository of memory, memory is all over and covers the entire brain. While this is true of brain-memory, it is equally true of mind-memory. While the brain-memory is concerned with the chronological or biological events, mind-memory is concerned with the psychological experiences associated with these events. Thus psychological memory belongs to the entire functioning sphere of the mind. And so for the understanding of the movement of the personal or the psychological time, the entire field of mind needs to explored. For the completion of the incomplete experiences, there has to come a complete cessation of movement in the entire field of the mind, and not just in a portion of it.

It is very often stated that, in the hustle and bustle of modern life, how can one find time to complete one's experiences? One has constantly to rush from one thing to the other where it is impossible to allot time for the completion of one's experiences. And yet it is the incomplete experiences of the many yesterdays that act as the cause of tension, stress and strain—the cause of the killer deseases of the modern age. The question of completing one's experiences is not a theoretical question, nor is it a question for some psychologists for their experimentation. It is a real question for all, for without its resolution it is impossible to know what healthy and creative life is.

The psychological or personal memory, caused by the incomplete experiences of the past, resides not merely at the conscious level, its habitat is mostly in the subconscious regions of the mind. In one's life there are constant pulls both at the conscious as well as at the subconscious level. It is these pulls that are the creator of numerous tensions and strains. It is these that do not allow any of the incoming experiences to be completed. And so there arise piles and piles of incomplete experiences. They do not permit one to look at life and its events with a totality of attention. All the time the attention is broken up. Thus, one meets life and its happenings with a completely fragmented attention. Mind is for ever interested in keeping psychological experiences incomplete, for thus alone can the continuity of thought live. It dreads the break in that continuity. And so in the continuing-thought process no psychological experience can ever be completed. In a non-psychological experience there is no hang-over, for there is no involvement of that factor of mind which demands continuity. There is the involvement of the thought process, but it is of a mechanical or mathematical nature. Here the event and the experience synchronize. It functions at the chronological level. When this happens, there is no psychological hang-over and so no creation, psychological tension or stress.

We have seen that psychological memory arises when there is non-synchronization between the end of the event and the end of experience. This is the ground in which psychological memory and psychological time come into existence.

But the question is: what sustains this psychological or personal memory? From where does psychological memory derive its sustenance? It is born out of a hang-over, but what is that which keeps it going? Why does not psychological memory fade away with the lapse of chronological time? Very often people say that time heals everything. But the fact of the matter is that it does not. The lapse of chronological time enables psychological memory to lie low, ready to jump up at the slightest pretext or excuse. Some happening, some gesture, a word, a faint signal stimulates the dormant psychological memory. It is ready to be stimulated, needing some excuse or the other. And so in the duration of time, it does not die, it exists in suspended animation. Some factor sustains it and is biding its time to come up sometimes in great fury. The question is: where does it reside in its comparatively dormant period ?

There have been cases when a person, thinking he is free from the tensions of psychological memory, experiences a jolt of his life when the same old tendency makes a sudden appearance, and that, too, at a time when this was least expected. Evidently, it had been lying low waiting to show its ugly head at any time, particularly when least expected.

It is, therefore, necessary to find out its hiding place so that it can be rooted out, freeing us from its dreaded incursions. Obviously, its hide-out is not at the conscious but at the subconscious level.

It is quite obvious that the incomplete experiences of the past have their hiding places in the process of continuity functioning both at the conscious as well as the subconscious levels. It is in this process that the psychological memory finds its maintenance and nourishment. The personal or psychological memory needs the ground of continuity in which to seek its fulfilment. One may ask: what is this ground of continuity? Obviously, it is the habit mechanism functioning within the consciousness of man. Habit is, indeed, the continuing factor, and so it is here that the psychological memory resides, with the piles of incomplete experiences seeking completion in time. Habit is the enormous field where this personal memory has its habitat and from where it exercises pull after pull demanding fulfilment. This field of habit is once again both at the conscious as well as the subconscious levels, more in the latter than in the former. And so, in our inquiry into the problem of self-transformation, we must needs explore this mysterious realm of habit, both conscious as well as subconscious.

8. *The Habit Mechanism*

EVERY unit of life seeks its biological survival and to this end takes security measures by building up suitable defence mechanism. This is but natural, for it must survive if it is to serve any useful purpose. Very often nature itself resorts to the method camouflage which enables the unit of life to protect itself against external dangers. Nature develops its own biological habits in order to provide for the survival of a particular species. This habit is its biological or physical heredity. Nature maintains its hereditary mechanism and within this heredity brings about structural changes which are known as variations. These are modifications in the outer structure of things. They do not constitute qualitative changes but only those that are concerned with outer forms. They do not suggest differences of kind but only of degree. They are modifications and are not mutations where the hereditary background is not disturbed but is kept intact. A mutation occurs only when the hereditary background is broken up. The units of life must have a certain amount of stability as otherwise their chances of survival are very remote. And yet nature sees to it that a unit of life maintains its adaptability in the midst of its stability. Stability and adaptability seem to be contradictory, for in adaptability there is involved a disturbance in the state of stability. And yet nature combines these two in a remarkable manner. If the unit of life cannot adapt itself to changed environment, then it must be wiped off. And nature does this relentlessly. It did not hesitate to wipe off even the giant dinosaures. Security and adaptability have been the two conditions laid down by nature for the propagation of the units of life. This constitutes nature's established habit.

Nature adopts this way, because in habit lies the factor of the conservations of energy. It is said that nature is careful of the type but careless of the single life. This may seem cruel so far as the functioning of nature is concerned. It is only through the preservation of the type that nature maintains the continuity of the life stream. In the habits of nature we see this inexorable pursuit of the factor of continuity. All variations and modifications arise in the field of continuity. But this continuity cannot be at the expense of the evolutionary process. And it is for this that it demands the characteristics of adaptability from the units of life that are protected by nature. Survival and security are guaranteed by nature but not at the cost of adaptability. This is the biological principle accepted by nature in its entire evolutionary game.

We are not, however concerned in this book with the biological security and survival in the field of evolution. Our main concern is at the psychological level. For here, too, the principle of evolution holds good.

We discussed in earlier pages that a unit of life can revitalize itself and regain lost energy, only if it constitutes a living or an open system and not a closed one. The closed system is a mechanical system where self-organization is not possible. But then does not habit-formation represent a closed system? In fact, there is nothing so closed as a habit. As we saw earlier, a habit represents a continuity process. Such a process is by no means open. In fact, habit becomes a mechanical movement, driven and maintained by its own mechanical laws. The defence mechanism created by habit must create a state of thermodynamic equilibrium. It would accelerate the running down process leading to death and extinction. If this be so, then habit is surely the anti-thesis of all process of renewal. We have seen that psychological or personal memory is sustained by habit. The personal memory demands a continuity of event and, therefore, the experience associated with it. It is out of a demand for continuity that habit is formed. Habit is the greatest defence mechanism that man and nature establish. Thus, it keeps out the incoming of new impulses and influences from life. Habit seeks to guard the hereditary factors, for thus alone continuity can be maintained. It may allow variations or modifications to arrive but certainly no mutations or fundamental changes. Thus, habit is a closed circle in which life moves covering the same ground again and again.

And yet, both biologically and psychologically, the unit of life must have security and survival. A child needs the security of the mother, otherwise it cannot live. For its survival, the protection given by the mother is absolutely essential. Without protection no unit of life can continue, it would be overpowered by the external forces of life. Habit not only maintains the continuity of life's existence, it supplies the mechanism by which energy is not frittered away, nay it is conserved. Thus, it saves the loss and dissipation of energy so very much needed for the survival of the unit of life. And yet by this very protective mechanism it brings into existence a closed system. And we have seen that a closed system must needs move towards its extinction with no prospect of regaining its energy.

We are, indeed, on the horns of a dilemma. Without the protective armour of habit a unit of life cannot survive, and yet habit, a creator of a closed system, offers no other prospect but of a total extinction of the self-same unit of life. To protect the unit of life in order that it may face its extinction—this seems to be the role of habit, whether biological or psychological. Since habit does not allow any fresh air to come in, the unit of life is given the prospect of a suffocating death, whether slow or fast. But without habit there is no continuity, and with habit there is extinction due to the state of thermodynamic equilibrium coming into existence. But then what is the way out?

Earlier we said that nature does protect a unit of life but expects from it a quality of resilience. Nature lays down a condition while supplying the protective armour for the security and the survival of the unit of life. This resilience is the quality of adaptability. Nature is ruthless in maintaining this condition, for it has no use for the unit of life that cannot adapt and re-adapt to the changing conditions of life. It demands the evolution of types that can quickly adapt to the geographical or other changes in the environmental conditions. It wants the unit of life to maintain its openness in the midst of all the protection and security supplied by nature. We have seen that in the formation of habit there is the survival of the hereditary factors. The maintenance of heredity is the guarantee for continuity. It is this factor which gives an assurance that the continuity of the species is not in jeopardy. The species may be biological or psychological. The continuity of the species or of the race is guaranteed because of this hereditary factor kept undisturbed. But then a habit leads to a condition of a closed circle. And adaptability demands a condition of openness. How can the two co-exist?

While discussing the question of equilibrium, we stated in the earlier chapters that three states need to be taken into account: the total equilibrium, the near equilibrium and the far-from-equilibrium. The far-from-equilibrium is a state of instability. The organism is far from a stable condition. It is in a condition of great perturbation, of tremendous disturbance. The condition of total equilibrium or what is known as thermodynamic equilibrium is a state of inertia where no movement is possible. It is on the threshold of death or extinction. It is in a condition of total entropy where the energy has completely ebbed out. But there is a middle state known as near-equilibrium which is as it were a stop-over between the two conditions. It is just an interval, a dynamic interval. It is a critical point or a bifurcation point. Nature, while producing mutations, seems to be acting at this critical point. It is out of the near-equilibrium ¦state that the far-from-equilibrium condition comes into being. But the condition is that the near-equilibrium state functions as a living and not as a closed system.

It is needless to say that the near-equilibrium state has still the quality of stability born out of the protective armour. And yet this stability has an element of elasticity or pliability. Stable and yet pliable is, indeed, the characteristic of the near-equilibrium state. If it is not pliable, then it will become a mechanistic and non-living system leading inexorably towards death and extinction. But if it is pliable but not stable, then its chances of survival would be very thin. If the unit of life has both stability and pliability, then it has the quality of openness which is the prerequisite for the self-organizing process to come into being. It is only here that mutations can take place. For here there is no rigidity of the organism, and yet it has the strength of survival due to the protective armour that surrounds it.

Writing about mutations, Julian Huxley, the eminent biologist says : '...spontaneous change or mutation of single factors has been and still is probably the most important source without which evolution could not take place.' Thus, mutation seems to be the other word for the emergence of a self-organizing process about which Prigogine speaks. However, mutation so far has been a mystery. As Julian Huxley says, the scientists do not know how mutations take place, they only study mutable organisms. In terms of the theory of Prigogine, there seems to be taking place the unravelling of the mystery of mutations. The story of how mutations take place seems to be unfolding itself through the self-organizing process at the critical point of far-from-equilibrium state. But this state can come only when stability and adaptability co-exist in an organism. Le Comte du Nouy, the French scientist, says in his book, *The Human Destiny*:

> It is not the being best-adapted to his environment who contributes to evolution. He survives but his better adaptation eliminates him from the ascendent progression, and only contributes to increase the number of more or less stagnant species that people the earth.

The near-equilibrium state may either proceed towards thermodynamic equilibrium or my move towards far-from-equilibrium depending upon whether the organism has the quality of stability alone or it has along with it the characteristic of elasticity too. At the point of the near-equilibrium state stablity and elasticity together constitute the livingness and the openness of that organism. This alone can take it to the far-from-equilibrium state where the self-organizing system emerges initiating the organism into a new order of existence. The near-equilibrium state is certainly a state of perturbation or fluctuation, of unease and discontent. Either this can move towards death and extinction or it can move towards a new order of existence. But this movement depends upon the co-existence of firmness and flexibility—if only the former, then the organism will come to a breaking point, if only the latter, then it will be swept away by the perturbation. They together can alone assure the organism to come to a breakthrough into a new order of existence.

We are essentially interested in the psychological aspect of this entire prospect of breakup or breakthrough. And so, at the psychological level, if there is built up the characteristic of firmness and flexibility, then the prospect of emerging into a new order, out of the utter chaos, seems very bright indeed. This shows a psychological make-up of confidence and hesitancy— the mesculine and the feminine aspect of consciousness. This is the way of life indicated by the bamboo in nature.

We have been discussing in this chapter the security and survival of the units of life. We saw that habit is the one instrument used both by man and nature to seek security and survival, for habit denotes a field of continuity. A unit of life feels secure only when the field of continuity prevails. It feels that it can survive only when continuity reigns. And since habit indicates the stream of continuity, all problems of security and survival centre round the sphere of habit. However, nature takes the precaution to warn the unit of life that its security can be guaranteed only if it shows forth the characteristic of flexibility so as to adapt itself quickly to changing environment. If this caution is not heeded, then the organism loses its chance of survival—it is wiped off and thrown uncremoniously on the discarded heap of failures.

While nature does this, man is unmindful of this caution. In the field of psychological living, where man essentially functions, this aspect of the co-existence of firmness and flexibility is lost sight of. When at the near-equilibrium state, if this requirement is lost sight of, then the organism moves towards a 'terminal' state from where there is no recovery possible. At the theremo-dynamic state of equilibrium, no choice is left for the organism, it must move towards its extinction. At the far-from-equilibrium state, there is a choice, but it lies with life or nature itself. It is only at the state of near-equilibrium that there is the possibility of choice, but this choice demands the co-existence of firmness and flexibility, the co-existence of masculine and feminine qualities. If these are not there, then the choice inevitably leads towards the extinction of the psychological species. And it is this which is the cause of the complete depletion of energy, the movement towards total inertia. At the near-equilibrium state the organism is aware of the perturbation—the disturbance. The organism is sensitive. This is not so at the state of total equilibrium. And because of the awareness of the disturbance or perturbation there is a livingness in the unit of life. This livingness is faced with the choice, but if the choice is in terms of firmness only, that is, in terms of the habit mechanism only, then the perturbation is bound to move towards a condition of total inertia. And this is what happens—it is the wrong choice that leads towards the terminal state, it is a state from where there is no return possible.

While in the movement of nature there is a saving grace, in the effort of man there is none. When we talk of the human being, the problem of survival and security is not so much biological as it is psychological. Man needs psychological security and survival. And for this he seeks a base of continuity. In this search he builds up habit mechanism at the psychological level. To save himself from psychological obliteration, he builds habit after habit. He becomes entrenched in habit. The habit is his defence mechanism. He clings to it as firmly as possible leaving no trace of flexibility. And it is the firmness of psychological habit that lands him into a terminal state, a state which is a point of no return. Medical men all over the world testify to one thing with regard to their patients they are prepared to swallow any number of pills but are unwilling to change their pattern of life. Very often a change in the pattern of life would soften the habit mechanism and a certain amount of flexibility would come into operation. And so in firmness and flexibility together, there may come about a change of a completely unpredictable nature. But this the patient is not prepared to do. He clings tenaciously to his pattern of habit, for, in the firm holding on to habit there seems to him the only way of security and survival. Most often it is this which leads him to extinction and end. But this is not the case merely at the bodily or biological level. It is more so at the psychological aspect of his being. Man does not build in his psychological nature that safe-guard which nature does at the biological level. And so in nature we see the movement from near-equilibrium state to far-from-equilibrium state where suddenly a new order of existence emerges. In the case of human beings, by and large, the near-equilibrium state moves on to thermo-dynamic equilibrium or to total inertia which is only the other word for death and extinction.

In the functioning of psychological habits, man builds up a strong machinery of reaction, for reaction being a chain supplies the element of continuity which man desires for survival and security at the psychological level. Through reaction man forges an instrument for continuity. But life, functioning at the psychological level where finer and subtler elements operate, the search for security is utterly elusive. That is why J. Krishnamurti says that psychologically there is no future, for here the flux of life is enormously rapid compared to the mechanical and mechanistic aspects of existence. And so here it is even more necessary to show forth greater flexibility and elasticity. There is greater need for tenderness and gentleness in dealing with psychological situations than in physical happenings. But such tenderness goes contrary to the firmness of psychological habits giving birth to reactive mechanism.

The strongest and the most powerful psychological defence mechanism forged by man is the reactive process. It is reaction that prevents fresh life impulse to penetrate the psychological armour created by man for survival and security. Man is ever afraid of a direct encounter with life. He feels that such a direct encounter would endanger his security. And so he prefers to live behind the walls of reaction. Now a reaction has its roots in the incomplete experiences of the past, and, therefore, it arises from the ground of psychological memory. It assures to man a psychological continuity. In the chain of reaction, man feels protected, for he feels that he will not be uprooted from the ground of continuity. Thus does reaction produce a closed system where there is no meaningful interchange between the unit of life and the environment. Being a closed system there is the dissipation of energy and, therefore, a running down of energy. It can never know the arrival of what the scientist Prigogene calls 'the dissipative structure', a structure which dissipates entropy. In the system created by the reactive processes of the human mind there is no escape from the downward movement of entropy.

In man's psychological make-up reaction is the other name for habit. The habit is so entrenched that reaction is the only response which man knows. The reaction may be pleasant or it may be unpleasant, but whatever form it may take is the expression of continuity. In a reactive process no break with continuity is ever envisaged. But it is only in the moment of discontinuity that a new impulse of life can be experienced. The reactive processes breathe of rigidity and over-confidence. Any gap in this reactive activity is resisted with fresh reaction. For reaction seems to be the only assurance to the unit of life that it survives.

Our psychological life is, by and large, a reactive life. There is an immediate reaction to any challenge from outside. There is no interval between challenge and response, for an interval is regarded as a danger spot. The unit of life fears that its very security will be threatened if an interval is given. And so immediate reactions make the closed system even more closed. Every reaction quickens the pace of the life movement towards extinction and death. It is the death of one's identity, for it is the well-established mechanism of reaction which gives to man his sense of psychological identity. And so in the reactive process there is place only for rigidity—here elasticity or softness has no place whatsoever.

We have seen that the unit of life, whether biological or psychological, needs security and survival. But only if habit allows rigidity and elasticity to exist together, then would the near-equilibrium state move towards the critical state of far-from-equilibrium where alone a new order of existence can come into existence. But mind is unable to envisage the co-existence of two contradictory factors of firmness and flexibility. Firmness is needed for the strength to survive, but this alone by itself leads to closed system. If the system can have protection and yet it is not too protected, then would arise the condition of flexibility. The firm and flexible like the bamboo—this, indeed, is needed for the arising of order of our chaos.

Why does not the mind envisage the existence together of the two seemingly contradictory elements? For this we must have a closer look at the nature and function of mind.

9. The Mind-Brain Syndrome

IT IS becoming more and more discernible in the modern world, in field after field of human interest, that reductionism has no validity in understanding the problems of life. In reductionism there is an effort to pin down everything to single factors. But nothing can be reduced to single causes of the fact of interrelationships. Nothing exists in isolation; everything is interrelated. In fact, physicists tell us that they see nothing but interrelationship. Prof. Eddington said years ago: 'The electron vibrates and the whole universe shakes.' This is no exaggeration. Over the years there has grown a Systems Theory which, in the words of Peter Russell in his book *The Awakening of the Earth,* says that 'nothing can be understood on its own'. Thus there are no singular factors or causes to which everything can be reduced. This is exactly what the word syndrome suggests. It speaks of the concurrent movement of things. Now in a concurrent movement two things exist together, and so in their co-relationship alone they can be understood. In separation they make no meaning. The two together form one. It is in this sense that we speak of the mind-brain syndrome. But for a syndrome there must exist more than one thing, for relationship presupposes an existence of more than one. A system or a syndrome has no meaning without this concurrent existence.

But this is exactly the difficulty in discussing the mind-brain syndrome. By and large, people, including those belonging to science faculties and those in the sphere of medicine, regard mind and brain as identical. They think that mind and brain are the same, and it is on this basis that all experimentation goes on. If mind and brain are the same, then it is meaningless to talk about mind-brain syndrome. There cannot be a syndrome if only one thing exists; for the syndrome to come into existence there must be more than one existence. We have said that, by and large, medical science has regarded mind and brain as identical, for most of the medical drugs are based on animal experimentation and the mind at that level is very rudimentary, if it exists at all. Not to take into consideration the factor of the human mind and to prescribe treatment based only on the effects on animal brains is, indeed, dangerous—and this has proved so. The mind of man exercises its own influence, and this must be taken into account when prescribing treatment for human ailments. But, for the consideration of this factor, there has to be a recognition that mind and brain are not identical. They are two and not one.

Are mind and brain two? If so, are they related? If they are related, what is the nature of this relationship? How does this relationship function? These are some of the questions that need to be considered. And this is exactly what has been partly done and that, too, with great excellence by Wilder Penfield in his most interesting and thought-provoking book, *The Mystery of the Mind*. In the very beginning of his treatise, Dr. Penfield poses two questions: 'Can the brain explain the man? Can the brain achieve by neuronal action all that the mind accomplishes?' The duality of the brain and the mind is being increasingly realized, but there are always diehards in all spheres—in science and medicine too—who are unable to see this duality. In fact there are three aspects of the problem that need to be borne in mind. These three are the brain, the mind and the consciousness. Just as brain and mind are not identical, similarly mind and consciousness, too, are not identical. Mind is just one function of consciousness, but to the question of consciousness we shall turn later in this book. For the present we are concerned with the duality of the brain and the mind. Dr. Penfield says in the above book that the brain is a computer and the mind is the programmer. This is certainly the best description of the role and the function both of the brain and the mind. Some writers have called the brain a bio-computer meaning a living computer. All man-made computers are digital in nature and function. The human brain is not a digital but an analogue computer. The difference between the two is brought out by Dr. Hubert Dreyfus in his book, *What Computers Can't Do*, thus:

> The distinction between digital and analogue computation is a logical distinction.... The essential difference between digital and analogue information processing is that in digital processing a single element represents a symbol in a descriptive language, that carries a specific bit of information, while in a device functioning as an analogue computer continuous physical variables represent the information being processed.

Thus, the man-made computer has to be fed by sequential inputs —the items of information given one by one—whereas the human brain, functioning as analogue device, accepts information all at once, not one by one. The brain receives information all at once not in a sequential manner. This is the great difference between the computer devised by nature. In creating this analogue computer of the brain, nature has worked wonders, John Pfieffer in his book, *The Human Brain*, says:

> Nature manages to perform her feats in exceedingly small spaces. Her vacuum tubes are microscopic cells, her fibres many times finer than the filaments of a spider's web. Dr. McMulloch points out that the Empire State building would not be large enough to house a computer with its many tubes as there are nerve cells in the brain—and it would take Niagara falls to supply the power and Niagara river to cool it.

If the brain is a computer and that, too, of the analogue variety, then the question is: how does it function? A computer is supposed to have information-gathering device. What is such a device so far as brain is concerned? And how does the brain process this information with which it is fed? In other words, what is the role of the brain and how does it discharge that role? Dr. John Pfieffer, the great brain specialist, says that after studying the brain in its various aspects there still remains a mystery and that is the mystery of the mind. He says that, in all the researches of the brain, the researchers have not come across an entity called the mind. Thus mind is not identical with the brain. The brain and the mind are different but not unrelated. In fact, they are closely related. They function together, and that is why mind-brain syndrome is a subject of tremendous importance to solve many a problem of medical science, particularly in the field of health and healing. But, apart from medical science, mind-brain syndrome needs to be considered for tackling many problems of life. But we must first see the information-gathering mechanism which the brain has at its disposal. Brain itself is a very complex organ, and the research about it goes on slowly. Leaving apart the whole brain, even its topmost part, the cortex demands a very long and elaborate inquiry. John Pfieffer says:

[Cortex] is the thickest and the most densely overgrown part of the cerebral jungle, containing regions as mysterious and inaccessible as vast streches of the earth were a few centuries ago. No single scientist or group of scientists can understand the whole cortex, and it may take years to explore an area no bigger than a postage stamp.

If the human mind is a mystery, the brain, too, is not less mysterious. The brain receives information from the functioning of the sense machanism. The senses are the reporters submitting information gathered from the outside world. But the senses do not send all that they gather; if they were to do it, then the brain would be smothered by the amount of information that is supplied. The senses themselves sort out the pieces of information as an efficient secretary to a minister would do. The minister cannot be bothered by all the many details of happenings in his department. Only a selected data is placed before the minister. This is exactly what the brain does. After such sorting out by each of the five senses, the stream of information goes to the brain. But here, too, unlike the digital computers, the brain receives all sense impacts all at once—not one by one. The impacts of the five senses are communicated to the brain simultaneously. In an article appearing in the *Book of Popular Science*, it is said: 'If, for example, one touches a finger to a hot stove, the hand is drawn away almost instantly. If,

however, one had to take time about what he should do, a very
severe burn would result before the hand could be pulled away.'
Here the senses have acted on their own without reference to the
brain. Thus, the senses work as good and efficient secretary to
the big officer that the brain is. The brain is, indeed, an analogue
computer inasmuch as it receives inputs simultaneously and not
one by one as in a digital way. The brain has a two-fold
avenues of information-gathering—one from the senses and the
other from the mind itself. But we will not consider here the
nature of the second avenue. Here we are considering only that
source of information gathering which is represented by the five
senses. The senses send sense impulses through their appropriate
channels, and out of these the brain formulates a percept. The
percept is born out of the processing device of the brain. Like a
computer, the brain does the processing of information. Will
Durant in his book, *The Story of Philosophy*, with reference to
the different messages sent by the senses with regard to an
object, says :

It is the raw crude beginning of experience, it is what the in-
fant has in the early days of its groping mental life. It is not
yet knowledge. But let these various sensations group themselves about an object in space and time—say an apple—let
the odour in the nostrils and the taste on the tongue, the light
on the retina, the shape revealing pressure on the hand unite
and group themselves about this thing—and there is perception.

Thus, it is the function of the brain to transform raw sensations into perception. The giving of shape and form is the task
of the brain. This is its role as a computer—the processing of
raw sensations and forging a percept by giving shape and form
to the sensations. The brain is, indeed, a computer, far more
efficient than the best of the man-made computer. It has been
rightly said that while the brain is like a computer there is no
computer like the brain. Its role and function is to process the
numerous sensations that arrive from the sense organs. But it is
not enough that the sensations are grouped in order to process a

percept. For future action, the computer needs to have the language of symbols. It would be a torture to use each time all material processed as a percept. The percepts would be too many. Just as the numerous sensations are processed for shape and form, the many percepts also have to be processed into symbols so that a symbol can call out the various percepts instantly. That is why a computer needs a symbol-language to do its work speedily and expeditiously. For here lies the value of a computer —its quick calculation. The computer does not have to go each time through the maze of perceptions, a symbol is enough. Each computer has its own language of symbols. It is this which is given by the mind. Out of the percepts it is mind that evolves a concept or a name. The name is, indeed, the symbol in all areas of relationship, whether with things or with persons or with ideas. When the name is uttered, it calls forth numerous percepts with reference to the relevant point of relationship. If the role and function of the brain is to give shape and form to sensations, it is the role of the mind, with reference to the brain, to assign names to percepts. We live in the world of name and form, and this has been fashioned by the joint effort of the brain and the mind. The mind has many other functions, but here we are talking of the role of the mind with reference to the role of the brain. There is, indeed, a mind-brain syndrome. They are different but closely related. If the brain and the mind function together, then there is no confusion in action, because right perception through name and form enables one to act rightly. It is the name with which the mind enables the brain to issue orders for action whereby senses are spurred into activity. But how is one to be sure that the mind has given to the brain for action the right name? If the name is wrong, then the action that emerges may not be right. John Pfieffer says: '...a computer can be designed to do anything you tell it to do. The only requirement is that you make your commands sufficiently specific and clear-cut.' The brain is not merely the organ of perception, it is also the organ for action. The various bodily organs begin to act always under the orders of the brain except those actions which the senses undertake to do such as the involuntary activities of the body like the heart-beats, breathing, digesting food etc. When an interference by the brain and mind in these involuntary activities takes place the bodily ailments appear. But, apart from these involuntary activities, the body moves at the behest of the brain. Who motivates the brain to act? It is the symbol with which the brain is fed that motivates it to issue orders to the organs of the body. If the symbols of the mind are indistinct or false, then the brain-orders to the body are bound to be defective. It is quite true that the brain is the computer, and it is the mind that is the programmer. It is the programmer that must release the symbols on the basis of which the brain can act. The efficiency of the computer alone is not enough, there has to be the absolute reliability of the programmer without which the end-result cannot be correct.

What do we mean by the reliability of the programmer? Who is the programmer? Dr. Penfield says rightly, that the mind is the programmer. The brain which is a computer like all computers, needs a programme which it can process out of sensations into percepts. But the programme has to have a programmer. While discussing the duality of mind and brain, we have to realize that there is a close relationship between the two, meaning thereby that each communicates with the other. The brain communicates with the mind through sensation-perceptions. But does the mind communicate with the brain? Obviously through a programme. John Pfieffer says: '...a computer can be designed to do anything you tell it to do. The only requirement is that you must make your commands sufficiently specific and clear-cut.' In order that the programme may be specific and clear-cut, the programmer has to be precise and exact. Now the programmer is the mind and so, if it is to be precise in its commands, it must be free from all its distractions. It must be free from all factors of conditioning. But this is exactly the difficulty in the functioning of the mind. For it experiences all the time the pulls of incomplete experiences of the past because of the motivations of the psychological memory. It is unable to display a totality of attention, and without this how can it perceive rightly whatever is presented to it? So for it, to be precise in its commands, seems to be an impossible proposition.

But apart from this, there is an inherent difficulty in the functioning of the mind which prevents it from becoming precise in its instructions—and, that is, that the mind is unable to perceive the whole. Its thinking is in opposites. In fact, all thinking is relational, and, therefore, it does not see anything by itself but only in relation to its opposites. Its perception itself is fragmented, and so precision is a condition difficult to fulfil. It is also driven hither and thither by likes and dislikes, by the pleasant and the unpleasant, and so all its commands and instructions are conditioned and coloured. If that be the case, the programmer itself is vitiated in its perception and, therefore, in its command. The brain may be very efficient, but it is subjected to orders that are confused and far from precision.

One may inquire as to how the mind communicates with the brain. The brain does by sensations-perceptions. But how does the mind carry out its work of communication? It does by mental formations or by mental images. Image is the language which the mind uses for its communication with the brain. The images have to be not only precise and clear but also true through right perception. But, for the perception to be right, there has to be a totality of attention and, therefore, the experiencing of the whole. In a fragmented perception, the vision of whole is lost. And so the image transmission is based on a fragmented perception. And the brain will process whatever it receives by way of image-transmission.

Mind is rooted in habit and, therefore, functions from the ground of habit. And the habits of the mind are deep-rooted. They are hard to die. These habits are in the form of mind's firm beliefs, opinions, and conclusions. Thus, through habit mind becomes a closed system. And a closed system has increasingly less and less energy at its disposal. An enervated instrument can hardly put vitality in the transmission. And so the image-message of the mind lacks vitality and, therefore, livingness. Needless to say, it is the whole that is alive, the part is devoid of life. This is so particularly at the psychological level where man abides more than at the biological level. And so how can the command that lacks life and vitality even have any effectiveness? The mind-brain syndrome is unable to function with any precision or effectiveness. There must come the perception of the whole. But how is one to come to such a perception, for unless this condition is fulfilled there can be no synchronization between the mind functioning and the functioning of the brain. And lack of synchronization leads to illness and disharmony. Health demands perfect synchronizations at all levels—biological, vitalistic, psychological and spiritual. But above all there must be the synchronization between the mind and the brain functioning. And health is, indeed, wholeness; we must, therefore, turn to the problem of wholeness, and this we propose to do in the next chapter.

10. The State of Integration

THERE is, indeed, a world of difference between synthesis and integration. The former is a construct of the mind. The mind, in order to understand anything, breaks it into parts. It can only proceed by analysis. That is the way of science and the way of intellect. It believes that without an investigation of a thing, part by part, it cannot understand what it seeks to investigate. This applies to all aspects of life, for the process of analysis is applied to things, to ideas and to human situations as well. Alvin Toffler says in his introduction to Prigogine's book *Order Out of Chaos* that

> One of the most highly developed skills in contemporary Western civilization is dissection: the split-up of problems. We are good at it. So good, we often forget to put the pieces back together again.
>
> This skill is perhaps most finely honed in science. There we not only routinely break problems down into bite-sized chunks and mini-chunks, we then very often isolate each one from its environment of a useful trick....In this way we can ignore the complex interactions between our problem and the rest of the universe.

We have been discussing in the last chapter about interrelationships because of which reductionism has no validity one cannot reduce everything to matter, nor can one reduce all things to mind. Mind and matter form a syndrome, and so one has to take into account the interrelationship. Those who follow the way of analysis and dissection say that, even though they break up a thing or an event or an idea into tiny parts, they do not end there. They tell us that they do not merely analyse, they also synthesize. Analysis and synthesis is the twin method they use. Yes, it is true that they do not merely break up, they also put back the broken parts into a whole. But there the question arises: what is a whole? F. Capra, in the introduction to his own book entitled *The Turning Point,* says that the whole is not the sum of the parts, it is greater than the sum of the parts. By putting the parts together the whole is not arrived at. The whole is not identical with the total.

These days we hear much about hologram or holographic device. It is a camera device by which one can have a many-sided or multi-sided view of an object. For example, if one is looking at a car under this holographic device, one would see all the parts of the car all at once—its front and its back, its top as also its bottom, its left side and right side together. This is what happens in the holographic device. But is this the perception of the whole? In normal observation things are seen one by one, in sequence. In the holographic device the various things are seen all at once. Writing about this device in his book *The Awakening of Earth,* Peter Russell says:

In a hologram...each point on a photographic plate records data about the whole image. Every part of the image is encoded in every part of the plate. When light of a particular kind is shone through the plate, the image can be made to appear, and it stands out from the plate as a three dimensional image. Since any region of the plate contains information about the whole image, it can give rise to the whole image. In this sense the image is enfolded throughout the plate.

This holographic device has arisen out of David Bohm's postulate regarding the implicate and the explicate order. It is suggested that the universe may be like a hologram, with the whole recorded in every part. However, David Bohm states:

This implicate order is never perceived directly. What we see is the explicate order, specific forms which are generated from the underlying implicate order. Ultimately...the entire universe has to be understood as a single undivided whole in which separate and independent parts have no fundamental status.

We shall comment later on the above statement that the implicate can never be perceived directly. What we perceive is the manifestation of the implicate order in the realm of the explicate order. But the explicate is fragmented into space and time as all manifestations are. And so if we see only the implicate manifesting in the explicate, then surely we are not seeing the whole. But we shall revert to this subject as to why the implicate order cannot be perceived directly. Here we are concerned to find what it is that is seen in the holographic device. Do we see the whole in the hologram?

It is true that in the hologram there is a many-sided or multi-sided view of things. But even the many-sided view is restricted to dimensions of space. However, nothing exists entirely in space. It is in space-time that all things and events exist. If the hologram shows the many-sided view in space, then surely it is not a whole view. There is the time axis involved in everything that exists. But the hologram has no means by which to show the time-view of things. A car seen from all sides is not the whole view of the car, for the car has existed in time also. But the hologram is unable to reveal the time-dimension of the car or of any object or event. This is a major drawback so far as the holographic view is concerned.

But let us suppose that this handicap is removed and we have a holographic device which shows all sides of space-time continuum. Even then can we say that we have the whole view of a thing or an event? By this device we can have the many-sided view in terms both of space and time, but is many-sided view the whole view? It is true that the many-sided view may give us the total view, total in the context both of time and space. But is the whole identical with the total? In hologram what is seen is the different parts together in space, not in time. But is whole the sum of the parts? The total indicates the sum of the parts. As F. Capra says: 'The whole is greater than the sum of the parts.' This indicates that the whole is not identical with the total. Even if the hologram shows all the parts of an object or an even in time as well space, the perception is not of the whole; it may at best be the perception of the totality of the aspects of the object or the event. The whole has to do with the implicate order, and David Bohm says that the implicate order cannot be seen directly. Only its manifestations can be seen in the explicate order. In the implicate and the explicate order we are dealing with the unmanifest and the manifest respectively. To speak of the unmanifest and the manifest as identical is utterly meaningless. They are different and yet closely related. What is the nature of this relationship? To know this is also to know the nature of relationship between the whole and the total.

How are the manifest and unmanifest, the explicate and the implicate related to each other? The unmanifest is in the manifest but not of it. By no dissection or analysis of the manifest can the unmanifest be found, and yet without the unmanifest the manifest would cease to exist. In the manifest the total can be found but not the whole, for the whole is greater than the sum of the parts. The total is made up of the sum of the parts. Thus, the whole is not the many-sided or the multi-sided view of things or events. The hologram gives the many-sided view, it may give the vision of the total but not of the whole. How is then the perception of the whole to be vouchsafed? But before we examine this question let us go to the beginning of this chapter.

We began the chapter with synthesis and integration. We said that synthesis is the construct of the mind. It is arrived at by the mind putting together the parts that emerge out of the process of analysis and dissection. Science and intellect do not merely analyse, they also synthesize what has been analysed. Analysis is the breaking up of an object, an event or an idea into constituent parts. But they do not leave the matter there. After examining various parts one by one, they put them together; and this is what is known as synthesis. But how is the work of synthesis done? By culling out the similarities comprising the parts. It is these similarities that are brought together by the human mind, and when this is done we declare that a synthesis has been arrived at. Naturally, in this process the dissimilarities are eliminated. But the original object, event or idea contained both the similarities and dissimilarities. They together constituted the livingness of the thing analysed. With the dissimilarities eliminated, the object, the event or the idea is divested of its living quality. And so the sythesis produces something utterly mechanical. It brings together the structure but misses the spirit. Thus, the synthesis can never give one vision of the whole—it is even less than the total.

It is in integration that the whole resides. The integrity of anything—maybe an object, a person or an event—indicates its wholeness. The whole is indivisible, for even in the tiniest part the whole exists. The whole has nothing to do with quantity; it is the quality, and surely quality can never be divided. In every part, even the smallest, the quality remains unchanged. The gold bar and the gold dust may differ in quantity, but they do not differ in quality. Both contain the same goldness. In integration there is the qualitative oneness; the two, even though quantitatively different, are qualitatively one. The manifest is full of diversity and manifoldness, the unmanifest is one and indivisible. To perceive quality in quantity is to see the whole in the part. And without the presence of the quality, any amount of quantitative progress and development is mere structure without the spirit. Thus, not in synthesis but in integration the quality of oneness can be discovered.

The quality is the wholeness, but this cannot be directly seen as David Bohm says. If it cannot be seen, then how does one know it? The quality is something intangible. It is in the part and the parts, but it is not of them. It is imperceptible, for it is only an intimation of the unmanifest in the world of manifestation. Without it the manifestation is lifeless. Without it the manifestation may be superb as a structure, but it is without the presence of the spirit. In one of the Upaniṣads, the *Kena Upaniṣad*, the teacher answers to the inquiry of the pupil who wants to know who moves the universe, who motivates life's activities. He wants to know who speaks, who hears, who thinks. The question of the pupil is:

Who sends the mind to wander afar? Who first drives life to start on its journey? Who impels us to utter these words? Who is the spirit behind the eye and the ear?

It is interesting to note that the young man does not want to know the how and the why of things, he wants to know the what—what is it that impels the speech to speak and the mind to think? In the Upaniṣad the teacher replies thus:

It is the ear of the ear, the eye of the eye, the word of the words, the mind of the mind, and the life of the life.

What is the ear of the ear and the eye of the eye—what is the mind of the mind? Is it something invisible? No, it is something intangible which cannot be held by any instrument of tangibility—and yet without it the ear cannot hear, the eye cannot see, the mind cannot think. But the pupil of the Upaniṣad wants to know what this is? To this the teacher replies by saying:

There the eye goes not, nor words nor mind. We know not, we cannot understand—how can we then explain—what it is?

The whole or the quality of things is not something that can be known and mentally understood. The whole cannot be known, but it can be felt, it can be experienced. The quality of things cannot be understood by thought, it can be felt and experienced. But how?

The pupils of Upaniṣads have been intrepid inquirers, not to be satisfied easily. This nature of relentless inquiry we find in Upaniṣad after Upaniṣad. The teacher says to the pupil that reality or that thich the pupil wants to understand is beyond the field of the known as far as the mind is concerned. It cannot come within the purview of mental or intellectual understanding. And he says to his pupil:

What cannot be spoken in words, but whereby words are spoken, know that alone to be Brahman, the Spirit—and not what people here adore. What cannot be thought with the mind, but whereby the mind can think, know that alone to be Brahman, the Spirit—and not what people here adore.

What cannot be seen with the eye, but whereby the eye can see, know that alone to be Brahman, the Spirit—and not what people here adore.

What cannot be heard with the ear, but whereby the ear can hear, know that alone as Brahman—and not what people here adore.

This is a very mysterious statement. It says that what the eye cannot see but without which the eye can perceive nothing, what the mind cannot think but without it the mind has no capacity to think—that alone is Brahman or Reality. The pupil wants to know what—he wants to know what Reality is. And the above is the answer of the teacher to the pupil. But the question still remains—how is this to be done?

But for this we must explore the depths of human consciousness...not the mind but the consciousness can provide the answer as to how Reality can be experienced. Reality is the whole, it is in the parts and yet not of them. The whole cannot be seen, it has to be experienced. It is the small silent voice of the intangible which can be heard not by the ear but by the ear of the ear, it cannot be seen by the eye but by the eye of the eye. What indeed is this? Not by dissection nor by analysis nor by synthesis can this be found. Its mystery lies in the stream of consciousness. Its depth and vastness must be explored, for neither the senses nor the mind has an answer to the question: what is Reality? And so we must do an exploration of the vast sea of consciousness in search of the answer to this question of questions.

11. The Stream of Consciousness

WE HAVE been discussing totality and wholeness in the last chapter and in that context we saw the perception given to us by hologram or by holographic devices. We saw that hologram cannot give us the perception of the whole. At best, it gives us the perception of the many-sidedness of things all at once, but this, too, in space, and not in time. But everything exists in space-time continuum. The hologram does not give us even an understanding of the total, because it leaves out the time factor. David Bohm who gave us the idea of hologram says, as quoted by F. Capra in his book, *The Turning Point*:

Bohm realizes that the hologram is too static to be used as a scientific model for the implicate order at the sub-atomic level. To express the essentially dynamic nature of reality at this level, he has coined term 'holomovement'. In his view the holomovement is a dynamic phenomenon out of which all forms of the material universe flow. The aim of his approach is to study the order enfolded in this holomovement, not by dealing with the structure of objects, but rather with the structure of movement, thus taking into account both the unity and the dynamic nature of the universe. To understand the implicate order, Bohm has found it necessary to regard consciousness as an essential feature of the holomovement and to take it into account explicitly in his theory.

Perhaps in the holomovement the missing factor of time may find its place but even then it will give us many-sided view of things and events as spread out in space and time. Bohm speaks of the structure of objects and the structure of movement. This latter aspect has the factor of time added to the otherwise static hologram model. But both space and time belong to the explicate order. They can give us the view of the total but not the whole. The whole cannot be seen, it can be experienced by faculty of consciousness.

But what is consciousness? One may say it is a faculty of awareness. And awareness denotes a subject-object relationship. The subject becoming aware of the object or an idea is consciousness. Now the subject-object relationship is not static. It differs from person to person, it also differs in the same person from experience to experience. Thus, awareness is intensely dynamic. And so holomovement demands an understanding of the nature and function of consciousness as awareness.

Consciousness is universal. Everything that exists has consciousness; whether it is dim or bright is a question of degree. Even the so-called inanimate stone has consciousness. Anything that responds, whether quickly or slowly, has awareness of the external impact of environment. It has to be noted that consciousness is the meeting place of the subject and the object, of the implicate and the explicate, of the unmanifest and the manifest, of the whole and the part. This meeting place is so dynamic that it continually moves on. And so an awareness of this meeting point demands a consciousness that is intensely sensitive. The meeting place is ever shifting, so rapidly shifting that the whole can be perceived in the twinkling of an eye or in the flash of lightning. One can look at Reality constantly but not continuously. Continuity is the sphere of mind and thought. Constant perception is possible only in the interval of discontinuity, only in the moment which is timeless. In the *Kena Upaniṣad*, the teacher says to the pupil who is eager to know Reality:

Brahman is unknown to the learned, and known to the simple.
Brahman is seen in nature in the wonder of a flash of lightning
—He comes to the soul—in the wonder of a flash of vision.

The flash of vision is momentary, and so Reality or Brahman can be experienced only in a moment, not in the duration of time. To be aware of the timeless moment is the secret of right perception where alone the whole is experienced, not in the totality of parts, not even in the re-assembly of parts in a synthesis. But this is exactly the difficulty of intellect or the faculty of logic and reasoning by which alone science moves. The difficulty of science is referred to by F. Capra in his book, *The Turning Point*. He says:

A science concerned only with quantity and based exclusively on measurement is inherently unable to deal with experience, quality or values. It will therefore be inadequate for understanding the nature of consciousness since consciousness is a central aspect of our inner world, and thus, first of all, an experience.... The more the scientists insist on quantitative statements, the less they are able to describe the nature of consciousness. In psychology the extreme case is given by Behaviourism, which deals exclusively with measurable functions and behaviour patterns and, consequently, cannot make any statement about consciousness at all, denying in fact even its existence.

Consciousness is an eternally dynamic phenomenon. It has not to be mistaken as identical with the mind. The mind is the function of consciousness and not the other way round as many scientists and psychologists seem to assert. The mind denotes in the initial stage a slowing down of the flow of consciousness, ultimately resulting in the formation of an island in the continuously moving stream of consciousness. The wholeness of anything can be experienced only in the moving stream of consciousness. In the duration of time the stream is sought to be broken up. When this is done, the living loses its quality of livingness. In Zen Buddhism, one of the Zen masters is supposed to have given a short instruction in the art of living when asked to do so, and he said, *Walk On, Walk On*. In the teachings of the Vedas also one finds the Vedic teachers asking the students— *Caraiveti Caraiveti*, meaning *Walk On*. It is only by walking on that life and its meaning and purpose can be comprehended. Since life for human beings is lived mostly at the psychological level, the above instruction *Walk On* must imply a ceaseless movement of the mind for comprehending life and its meaning. But then, it may be asked, is this not what human beings do all the time? The minds are ever active and challenging without hardly a stop. But can this continual movement of the mind give us life's understanding? If not, what is the meaning of *Walk On*. It is true that mind is continually on the move which means that there is non-stop movement of thought, but then the movement of thought is all the time out-of-step with the flow of consciousness. The movement of thought is a motivated movement under the pressure of mind's psychological memory with the ceaseless demand of the incomplete experiences of the past needing completion. And so the movement of thought is not in harmony with the movement of life. And so it is only when the movement of the mind ceases that the movement in the mind begins. It is the latter movement which is in synchronized harmony with the flow of consciousness. And so *Walk On* is possible only when the mind stands still. Then in this flow of consciousness can Reality, Truth or whatever one wants to call it, be experienced? The perception of the whole is vouchsafed to man only when the flow consciousness is seen in the background of mind's stillness.

Why does not mind move in step with the flow of consciousness? This is so because the mind moves under the motivation of likes and dislikes; it lingers and tarries and it is thus that it forms island after island in the ever-flowing stream of consciousness. The mind can perceive an object and an event or an idea by holding it. The stream of consciousness moves on and what is held by the mind is not Reality but its shadow, its memory. It is this which mind seeks to dissect and analyse, and, in the words of Dr. Alexis Carel, the mind of man wants to understand the living by dissecting the dead. And so it is not the consciousness held as a prisoner by the mind that can reveal the face of reality. The consciousness freed from the clutches of the mind can alone experience Truth, Reality or Wholeness.

But is there a consciousness other than that which operates within the confines of the mind? Are not mind and consciousness identical? It has to be understood that mind is neither the beginning of consciousness nor is it the end of consciousness. Modern physics tells us that the basic stuff of the physical universe is not matter, it is consciousness. But it is unable to say clearly and definitely what consciousness is. Keith Floyd suggests in his book, *Of Time and the Mind*, that the riddle of consciousness is unique, for 'consciousness itself is the only tool we have to examine consciousness'. There is a confusion here between consciousness and mind. Here it is stated, in an implied manner, that consciousness and mind are identical. Mind is involved in all acts of perception, and in the very act of perception it modifies the object of perception. This is becoming increasingly recognized in modern physics. Then how can the mind perceive what is. One cannot postulate an independent and an impersonal observer, and every observer is a participator. Keith Floyd says that the scientists cannot see what they want to see because 'that which they are looking for is that which is looking'. How can the perceiver see himself? But here we have to take into account various layers of consciousness. Mind is only one layer of consciousness. But it is not the only layer. Mind is one avenue through which consciousness perceives. If consciousness is awareness, then the history of evolution says that the point of awareness is not static, it is ever shifting. There was a time when mind had not come on the evolutionary scene. Consciousness was not functioning from the point of intellect which is at present the operating instrument of the mind. Animals are guided by instinct. Migratory birds fly thousands of miles away from their nests under the instruction of their instincts. And instincts serve them as unfailing guides. Even early humanity was guided by instincts. Men and women belonging to early aboriginal tribes could find out the right direction even in the midst of storm. In instinct the guidance is from the memory of nature. But in the history of evolution we see the arrival of intellect too, and men and women of this civilization are particularly dependent upon the guidance given by intellect. In intellect, too, there is the guidance of memory, but not the memory of nature, not the biological memory but the memory of the human mind which is by and large psychological or personal memory. In this memory there is the intervention of likes and dislikes, of the pulls of the incomplete experiences of the past. At this point the stream of consciousness is interfered with by the mind's activity in terms of lingering and tarrying or even of hurrying from the unpleasant aspects of personal memory. Thus, it is that mind superimposes on the stream of consciousness the flow of personal memory. But in the flow of two streams there is no harmony. Here, there has taken place a shift of consciousness from instinct to intellect. In this shift there comes into being a successive awareness because of the movement of psychological time superimposed on the flow of biological time. In instinct there is just the flow of time in terms of chronological time. It is in intellect that the factor of succession comes in. At the level of instinct, just the chronological present is the centre of awareness. At the level of intellect, the succession from past to future creeps in, and here the situation is still more complicated because of the factors caused by the movement of personal time. In any case, from instinct to intellect denotes a shift of consciousness. And so consciousness is not static, there are shifts in its flow. If so, there is no reason to believe that there cannot be further shift from intellect to that which is beyond the intellect. If consciousness is awareness, there are grades of such awareness, perhaps culminating in self-awareness where the mystery of the observer looking at himself too can be resolved. These grades of awareness are fully discussed in Eastern Psychology as indicated in the *Māṇḍūkya Upaniṣad*, one of the major Upaniṣads. There is the awareness of the conscious mind spoken of as the *jāgrita* of the waking state, the awareness of the subconscious mind known as *svapna* or the dream state, the awareness of the unconscious mind known as the *suṣupti* or the deep sleep state, and there is the awareness of the transcendental consciousness known as *turīya* state. These are differing states of awareness. As a shift takes place, there is a movement of awareness from point to point. Consciousness denotes a relationship between the subject and the object. In the shifting states of consciousness, there is, thus, a shift of awareness. And so there is no reason to believe that mind is the only instrument of awareness, of perception. Consciousness has to be understood in terms of this shifting awareness leading up to self-awareness where the observer sees himself in the mirror of life.

But how does this shift take place? Is it completely subject to external factors or to whims of nature? In fact, this shift can be consciously manipulated so that the flow of time can be hastened or can be slowed down but this demands the removal of the obstructing activities of the mind. The mind interferes with the flow of consciousness by erecting island after island in the vast sea of consciousness. To manipulate the flow of consciousness suggests the understanding of the technique of Yoga, for Yoga is the speeding up of the flow of consciousness; and that which can cause speeding up can also cause the slowing down. But this slowing down or speeding up is not by diverting the flow into directions that are against the very nature of the flow—this is what the mind does. But there is a hastening and a slowing which is in harmony with the natural flow of consciousness, not working at cross-purpose but with the intrinsic flow of consciousness itself. How is this hastening and elowing of the flow of consciousness possible?

We have been discussing the question of the vision of the whole. We have seen that the whole is greater than the sum of the parts. But is the whole away from the parts? It is in the parts and yet it is not of them. But if the whole is in the parts, then why does not one see it? It is because of the impediments put in the stream of consciousness. Due to these impediments, the consciousness becomes opaque. It must be rendered transparent so that the flow goes on without any obstruction. For this there must take place a conscious manipulation of the flow, not by the mind, for it invariably puts obstacles and impediments, but by a further shift of consciousness from intellect to insight or intuition. There has to be a two-fold shift—one of the extension of consciousness and the other of the expansion of consciousness. We must explore this two-fold movement.

12. The Living Tradition

THE controversy with regard to mind-versus-matter which raged vigorously in the scientific world during the nineteenth century seems to have abated. In fact, it is mind-over-matter which is gaining more and more ground. In ancient India, saints and sages said that mind is the cause of man's bondage and also the cause of his liberation. In one of the Upaniṣads it is said that the whole world is nothing but an expression of consciousness. Now consciousness is becoming more and more the subject matter of discussion in scientific and intellectual circles. Since matter has ceased to be material, attention has been shifted to the study of and investigation into the realms of consciousness. We have seen that consciousness is awareness, and this awareness covers a wide range from the little stirrings in inert matter to self-awareness in a human individual. Because of fluctuations in awareness or consciousness, the attention of the intellectual world is moving more and more from pattern to process, from structure to rhythm. In nature there is rhythm in all its movements. F. Capra says in his book, *The Turning Point*:

In the future elaboration of the new holistic world, the notion of rhythm is likely to play a very fundamental role. The systems approach has shown that living organisms are intrinsically dynamic, their visible forms being stable manifestations of underlying processes. Process and stability, however, are compatible only if processes form rhythmic patterns —fluctuations, oscillations, vibrations, waves. The new systems biology shows that fluctuations are crucial to the dynamics of self-organisation. They are the basis of order in the living world—ordered structures arise from rhythmic patterns.

There is evident more and more in the scientific world, a shift from structure to rhythm. There is this rhythmic factor seen in the functioning of consciousness as well. While the explicate order shows forth the element of structure, it is the implicate order which imparts the quality of rhythmic fluctuations to the manifest order. While structure represents a factor of continuity, it is rhythm that introduces the element of intervals of discontinuity. If structure does not respond to rhythm, then it becomes dead and sterile; it is rhythm that gives to it a quality of livingness. We saw earlier that evolution is discontinuity in the midst of continuity. Without the factor discontinuity the organism would move to rigidity of structure and, therefore, to its extinction. It is in rhythm that the factor of self-organization can become manifest, for, in the interval, which a rhythm indicates, there arrives the new impulse generating the self-organization process. Thus, rhythm is the secret of evolution.

In terms of consciousness, this rhythm implies the intensification and slowing down of the stream of life. A mere intensification or rapidity of the stream denotes a factor of continuity, similarly a slowing down of the current of consciousness also indicates a state of continuity. It is only in the alternation between intensity and slowness, which is the characteristic of rhythm, that the quality of livingness abides. This interval is the timeless moment in which alone Truth, Reality or Wholeness can be experienced. Consciousness is able to function in a healthy manner so long as this rhythm is maintained. It is when the rhythm is broken that illness of the body and of the mind starts. It is mind that breaks this rhythm of nature and desires to impose on the rhythm of life its own rhythm. Life functions happily so long as the rhythm functions without any interruption. The rhythm of life is described in numerous ways; in Chinese philosophy it is known as Yang and Yin, in Hinduism it is known as Śiva and Śakti. Modern psychology speaks of the masculine and feminine qualities of consciousness. This rhythm is the living tradition of life.

There is a rhythm of consciousness and there is the rhythm of mind. The former is the natural movement of life, while the latter is a movement imposed upon the natural movement of life by the operations of the mind. Obviously, they are in conflict, and it is this which is the cause of tensions, stresses and strains. The rhythm of mind is motivated by likes and dislikes, by the impulsions of the psychological memory. In this rhythm, too, there are the factors of continuity and discontinuity. But mind's discontinuity is no discontinuity at all; it displays the factors of continuity which are overt and those which are covert. It is continuity on a low key. It is more in the nature of respite from where to pursue the process of continuity with greater vigour. Mind wants its rhythm to prevail and so seeks to control the movement of consciousness. All that it succeeds in doing is putting up a barrier of obstruction to the onward movement of consciousness. Thus it is that it creates a condition of stagnation which it mistakes for security. And so it creates a closed system where no self-organization is ever possible. In a living system fluctuations are moments of creative instability from where a new order emerges. In such a system fluctuations or perturbations are the pointers of a breakthrough. In closed or mechanistic systems they are the heralders of doom and destruction.

How to get out of this predicament? As F. Capra says, as quoted in the earlier passage, stability and process are compatible. This is the rhythm of nature like particle and wave, like movement and stillness as depicted in the beautiful Hindu statue of Natarāja or Dancing Śiva. This is the supreme rhythm of life. But how is one to be free from the rhythm of the mind so that the natural rhythm of life may come into being? The rhythm of life expresses itself through consciousness, and it is this that we are trying to understand. Rhythm is, indeed, the secret of healthy living. Even in such a mundane field as military manoeuvering, rhythm of conquest and consolidation has to be maintained. An army cannot just go on conquering new territories. It has also to consolidate what it has conquered, otherwise the conquered territories may be seized by the enemy. Aggression and consolidation have to be the rhythm of the army that is on the march. Thus, speeding up and slowing down the rhythm of life has to be followed in all walks of life. But this speeding up and slowing down has to be not in terms of the rhythm followed by the mind, but in terms of the rhythm of life itself. But how is one to follow the rhythm of life when the mind is all the time superimposing its own rhythm?

There has come down through the ages a living tradition, particularly in India, to maintain this true rhythm of life, not getting entangled in the rhythm of the human mind. This is the tradition of Yoga and Tantra. Although they are different, they are not contradictory as is commonly supposed. We have seen that the rhythm of consciousness is the process of speeding up and slowing down. This is the masculine and the feminine aspects of consciousness. In terms of Hindu psychology, Śiva is the masculine aspect of consciousness even as Śakti is the feminine counterpart. They represent the conquest and the consolidation phases of consciousness, and both must exist if there is to be health and wholeness.

This rhythm is the age-old tradition expressed by Yoga and Tantra. Yoga is obviously the masculine expression even as Tantra is the feminine. In Tantra it is Śakti aspect of life that is worshipped signifying its emphasis on the feminine expression of life. Yoga is concerned with the conquest of new realms of being whereas Tantra is concerned with the aspect of consolidation, for it is the mother or the feminine aspect that looks after consolidation of the movement of life. Modern science has recognized the masculine and the feminine as the basic facts of life's expressions at all levels. In a sense, the particle and the wage represent the basic aspects of this phenomenon. It is mind that breaks this rhythm for the purposes of its own security. It can feel secure only in the unbroken state of continuity. Any indication of discontinuity is resisted by it vigorously, for discontinuity is the emblem of death and destruction for the mind. It is in this search for security that it follows the path of stagnation and extinction, for without the moments of discontinuity no fresh impulse can ever enter the process of life. But the question is: how to halt this action of the mind so that the vitality and the freshness of the rhythm of life can be maintained?

It is here that Yoga and Tantra are of inestimable value. It is Yoga that indicates the process of psychological conquest even as Tantra signifies the phenomenon of consolidation. For health and wholeness of the individual life the co-existence of these two processes is absolutely necessary. It is true that mind creates impediments in the even flow of the rhythm of life. But the mind cannot be bypassed. It is with the help of the mind that the mind can be transcended. In the practice of Tantra it is this aspect of one's inner discipline that is taken into account. Yoga may lose itself in aspirational speculation even as Tantra may get lost in mere technicality. It is true that Yoga is concerned with scaling new heights of consciousness and Tantra is concerned with consolidating each base so that the conquering team may return to its base as and when required. In the journey of life, too, conquest and consolidation must function together. Needless to say, in conquest it is the speeding up process that is evident whereas in consolidation it is the slowing down technique that is visible. Yoga by itself may result in sterile idealism whereas Tantra by itself may result in meaningless skills of technique. The latter is very much visible today where purposeless and utterly meaningless psychic developments are sought after. And so Yoga and Tantra must function together, for they constitute the natural rhythm of life and consciousness. While Yoga is the goal-setter, it is Tantra which is the energy-restorer. Obviously, both are necessary in the journey of life. Life becomes meaningless if there are no goals to be achieved, no new heights to be scaled. Life becomes frustrating if there is no continual restoration of lost energy. In the process of living, energy is bound to be expended, but there must be the means to regain lost energy. Yoga is, indeed, a speeding up process and Tantra is a slowing down process, for consolidation needs the operation of a slowing down phenomenon.

We have been talking of the non-synchronization of the rhythm of life or consciousness and the rhythm of the mind. A rhythm has intervals of discontinuity in the midst of continuity. But is there a moment of discontinuity in the movement of the mind? To talk of rhythm without an interval of discontinuity is to indulge in something meaningless. An interval of discontinuity is the very soul of rhythm. In the so-called rhythm of the mind an interval of discontinuity is consciously created, for the activity of the mind is always motivated. Mind attempts to slow down from the speeding up process only out of sheer exhaustion.

The moment of exhaustion is not an interval of discontinuity. It is a moment of suppressed continuity or may be a state of modified continuity. But modified continuity is not discontinuity. And so in mind's rhythm there is no interval of discontinuity, for the mind is for ever frightened of discontinuity regarding it as death. And so the so-called discontinuity of the mind is only an interruption of the ceaseless continuity in which alone mind finds its security. Its security is no more than a continuity functioning in a covert manner biding its time to operate with greater zeal.

And so it is not the question as to how the rhythm of the mind and the rhythm of consciousness could synchronize. The question is to stop the movement of the mind so that the natural rhythm of life may operate without any interruption or obstruction caused by the movement of the mind. We have said earlier that mind cannot be bypassed, and mind's approach to all situations and problems is binary which means the approach of either/or. And so in the approach of the mind the way is either to struggle or to submit. Our problems are to stop that movement of the mind in order that the rhythm of consciousness flows unobstructed. Can the problem of the mind be dealt with by the either/or process, that is, through struggle or submission? It is quite evident that by submitting to the ways of the mind there can be no relief. But what about struggling against the ways of the mind? Surely, this is what man has done through the ages but without success. Our concern is to stop the movement of the mind. Can this be done by fighting the ways and inclinations of the mind? The usual ways of spiritual life suggest that we must carry on a relentless war against the tendencies of the mind. Here the effort seems to be to bring the mind forcibly to a stop. But can mind be stopped by force? The Buddha once said to his disciples: 'If you tie the horse, then it will be even more restless'. But, then, what is to be done? Should the horse be let loose and allowed to wander wherever it likes? If neither of these, then what?

There is a third way and that is to transcend the mind with the help of the mind, to come to the quiet of the mind with the help of the mind. This is what Tantra indicates, for it has always suggested that one can convert the obstacles into stepping stones to rise higher. To fight the obstacles at the psychological level is a frustrating process. But to make use of the obstacles and impediments as instruments for spiritual ascent—this is what Tantra has suggested. In Tantra it is the very thought process that is used for transcending thought. In the whole approach of Yoga and Tantra, one is dealing with the reversible and the irreversible phenomena of life. Yoga is concerned with the irreversible even as Tantra is concerned with the reversible. Physical science today speaks of the co-existence of determinism and chance. In Yoga and Tantra we are faced with the co-existence of two seemingly contradictory factors. While Yoga deals with the speeding up process, it is Tantra that deals with the slowing down process. There is the arrow of time, but there is also the reversal of time. The reversal of time denotes the slowing down process. The arrow of time indicates the speeding up for an arrow speeds up in its ownward journey. We must go into the reversible and the irreversible processes as we explore the technique of Yoga and the discipline of Tantra.

13. The Hidden Variable

IN THE eighteenth discourse of the *Bhagavad Gītā*, Lord Śrī Kṛṣṇa, while expounding the theme of action to Arjuna, says that all actions have a five-fold cause, and this is true of every action without exception. The first among this five-fold cause is the ground from which the action emerges. The Sanskrit word is *adhiṣṭhānam* meaning a base or a ground. This ground is the motive which impels the action to take place. Then there is the actor. The third is the instrument of action, and the fourth is the pattern or patterns of action. This fourfold description of the causes of action is easy to understand. But the Gītā mentions the fifth aspect of the cause of all actions and that is *daivam*. This may be interpreted as divine intervention or something unknown and unpredictable. It is this that completely upsets the operation of the other four. This factor has been recognized in the researches of modern physics. The physicists speak of the local variables and the hidden variables. These two denote the existence of the predictable and the unpredictable factors operating at all levels of life's manifestation. The local variable can be predicted but not so the hidden variables. We are told that, while at the macroscopic level prediction in terms of probability is possible, no such prediction is possible at microscopic level. The hidden variable is the unknown and, therefore, the unpredictable. It appears from nowhere at any time and in any form. The predictable and the unpredictable are not two distinct phenomena. They are interlinked, integral part of every phenomenon. They speak of the operation of law and yet something that cannot be put in the framework of law. As Henry Stapp, the scientist, said: 'The theorem of Bell proves in effect, the profound truth that the

world is either fundamentally lawless or fundamentally insepar-
able.' Nothing in the world can be isolated from other things.
It is true that one cannot know anything unless one knows
everything. It is only when one looks at things in separation
that the paradox of law and lawlessness appears. But in nature
and in life there is no paradox, for here two seemingly opposite
things exist together. There is a complementariness between the
so-called two. But to comprehend the contradictory as comple-
mentary requires a shift in consciousness—from the successive
consciousness to the simultaneous consciousness. But this once
again brings us to the question of Yoga and Tantra.

The predictable and the unpredictable naturally bring us to
the question of the reversible and the irreversible time. It is
obvious that the reversible denotes the factor of predictability.
It is a part of the operation of law. The reversible is that which
can be called back, and this, indeed, is so with regard to that
which is predictable. The predictable is within the purview of
the law of probability. But the moment we say something is
probable, we suggest that it is not certain. Heisenberg's principle of uncertainty is all-pervading, meaning thereby that the
unpredictable is in the bosom of the predictable. And that is
why it is known as the hidden variable. The irreversible is within the reversible as the unpredictable, not away from the
predictable. That is why one reads in the *Bhagavad Gītā*, Srī
Kṛṣṇa telling Arjuna that all actions are rooted in the five-fold
cause, and *daivam* is a part of this five-fold cause. The fifth
cannot be isolated from the other four. In fact, the fifth seems
to be the overriding factor governing the five-fold cause. In the
Katha Upaniṣad, the Lord of Death tells his pupil: 'The eternal
is in the transient and the living is in the inanimate.' To the
mind of man this seems unbelievable. How can the two exist
together? And yet this is a fact that operates in all manifestation of life—there is a movement in stillness and a stillness in
the movement itself. It is here that Yoga and Tantra come to
our aid, for Yoga deals with the problem of stillness, and Tantra
is concerned with movement. It may be said that, while Tantra
is concerned with the reversible, it is Yoga that deals with the
problem of the irreversible· Although Yoga and Tantra cannot

be separated, we will consider them separately so that the intellect can grasp their essential teachings clearly.

Yoga and Tantra both deal with the working of human consciousness. Man's immediate problem is with the reversible and the predictable. This is so because he is for ever concerned with regaining the energy which he loses in the act of living. Unless he is able to deal with the problem of the renewal of energy, he cannot proceed further in life. He gets caught in the crisis of energy from which he is unable to step out. Is there a reversible process by which energy lost can be regained? Can man control the movement of time? For it is in the movement of time that energy gets dissipated. Is there another time apart from what is known as the arrow of time? In nature one sees that other aspect of time, for there is a continual process of reversal in nature shown in the movement of seasons, in the cycle of day and night, in the appearance of ebbs and tides in the flow of the seas, and in many other factors. Nature shows that in spring everything gets renewed even though winter had denuded all that was vital and living. But man does not experience this renewal and revitalization in his process of living. For him a thing is gone and gone for ever. The happy moments have gone in the limbo of the past never to be recovered. Is the law for man different from the law that operates in nature? Why can man not have the cycle of seasons if other forms of nature can have?

Although man regards himself as separate from and somewhat superior to nature, life has provided him with certain powers of which he is not aware and which, therefore, are not being used by him. These powers enable him to work with nature at a point higher than where other forms of life function. Either he uses these powers to help nature and work on with her, or he uses them to run counter to nature's ways. If he follows the latter path, then he experiences for himself woe and suffering· Nature is willing to accept man as a collaborator, but never as a competitor. Nature is willing to reveal her secrets to man if he will co-operate with her. H.P. Blavatsky says in her *Voice of the Silence* :

Help Nature and work on with her, and Nature will regard thee as one of her creators and make obeisance. And she will open wide before thee the portals of her secret chambers, lay bare before thy gaze the treasures hidden in the very depths of her pure virgin bosom.

If man would use the powers he has in co-operation with nature, then he will discover the secrets that lie within his own consciousness. Man possesses two-fold power which he has rarely used or when used he has sought to move counter to the ways of nature. By using these powers he can know the secrets of the process of the reversal and the irreversal within his consciousness. These powers are indicated in Yoga and Tantra.

But what are these powers? They are the formative power of thought and the directional power of consciousness. Earlier we have mentioned that mind and consciousness are not identical, they are different and yet closely related. The formative power of thought has to do with the functions of the mind even as the directional power of consciousness has to do with that which transcends the mind. While Tantra is concerned with the formative power of thought, it is Yoga that is concerned with the directional power of consciousness. These two must work together as otherwise man will face dire consequence. When the work of the two does not synchronize, man moves rapidly towards his degeneration and decay. This is borne out by the history of religious movements, specially in India. Tantra implies technique, method or process. But a technique by itself is meaningless, nay, even dangerous. It must have a purpose, right purpose, otherwise what we see today is bound to happen where we have nuclear technique but no clear formulation of purpose. Tantra represents Indian psychology—we say Indian because there are Hindu Tantra and also Buddhist and Jain. While Tantra gives us the basis of Indian psychology, it is Yoga which indicates the best in Indian philosophy. If philosophy and psychology do not function together, then both become sterile. Psychology without philosophy is purposeless even as philosophy without psychology is powerless. It is this which demands the need for the synthesis of Yoga and Tantra, in fact, this has become the supreme need of the modern age of science and technology.

We saw earlier that it is in the non-syncronization of the event and the experience that all problems of psycho-somatic illness arise, and by and large, the illnesses of the modern age are psycho-somatic. Man must first get rid of the symptoms of illness before he begins to reap the fruits of health. The whole problem of man's illness and health has negative and positive aspects. And it is in the synthesis of Yoga and Tantra that we are enabled to deal with the whole problem, negative as well as positive, about man's well-being. Tantra deals with the restoration of energy even as Yoga deals with the purposeful use of the restored energy. Their operation has not to be one after the other, they must function together simultaneously. That is why they involve the discovery of a new base of consciousness.

There are two aspects of Tantra, one psychic and the other psychological. Most often it is the psychic aspect that is unfortunately emphasized. Here the aim is to develop psychic or supernatural powers. This has led to the emphasis on developing the eight-fold psychic accomplishments, the *aṣṭasiddhi* as they are called. Here the effort is to solve the problem of energy loss by the development of psychic powers. And that, too, without solving the problems of frustrations and inner disharmony. It is the inwardly broken man that wants to have more and more powers. It is like the modern civilization, in a state of complete disharmony regarding the field of human relationship, wanting to have more and more nuclear powers to establish one's supremacy over the other. Today we see Tantra divorced from Yoga in all fields of life.

We have been discussing in this chapter the predictable and the unpredictable which are described as the *Daivam* in the Bhagavad Gītā. It is here that Tantra and Yoga can be of inestimable value. For Tantra, enables one to move consciously in the field of the predictable, and Yoga prepares him for the arrival of the unpredictable. By and large, man is afraid of the arrival of the *Daivam* or the unpredictable. He is afraid of the arrival of the unknown. But the fact of the matter is that it is only in the *daivam* or the hidden variable that nature or life indicates the right direction in which to move when one is caught in a crisis, when one is at the bifurcation point. But he cannot welcome the arrival of the hidden variable, the *Daivam,* so long as the field of predictable, the Local Variable, has not been explored, and that, too, not by remaining at the mercy of nature but by consciously expediting the process of the exploration of the field of the known. It is only when the field of the known with regard to any situation is explored as fully as possible that man is in a position to welcome the arrival of the unknown. The exploration of the field of the known and the experiencing of the arrival of the unknown—this is done by Tantra and Yoga respectively. But this requires moving away from the Tantra of psychic development to the Tantra of psychological fulfilment.

It is in the Tantra for psychic development that one gets absorbed by the question of the awakening of *kuṇḍalinī*—the dormant biological energy. And in the modern world, where man is frustrated by the dissipation of energy, there is an ever-increasing interest in the awakening of this dormant energy. Man wants more and more energy as otherwise he feels powerless to deal with the problems of life. But more energy for what? Is it for the pursuing of meaningless existence or is it for overpowering the other so as to gain supremacy in the competitive field of modern life? One must have the guidance of right philosophy, so that added powers do not lead to destruction and decay but to the enrichment and true fulfilment of life. But right philosophy is not the product of the mind. It is born when the touch of the unknown comes. But the touch of the unknown cannot be experienced unless one has explored the field of the known and the predictable. It is because of this that Tantra and Yoga must function together so that the mind is ready to learn, after the exploration of the known, and receive the arrival of the *daivam*—the hidden variable—as and when it comes.

Standing at the critical point of life, mind cannot show the right direction in which to move. It is in the arrival of the unknown that the right direction is found. But the unknown arrives only in a living and an open system of life, and that, too, not by waiting for nature to announce such an arrival but by consciously exploring the field of the known and the predictable.

How does Tantra do it? What are its instruments by which it consciously explores the field of the known and the predictable, thus expediting the work of nature? In the process of exploring the field of the predictable, does it bring the human consciousness to a point where the limits of the mind are reached bringing one to the very frontiers of the realm of intellect? Tantra for psychism and Tantra for exploring the field of human psychology—these two are its fields. By and large, it is the former that is pursued while the latter is completely overlooked. It is by the exploration of the latter field that the experience of the hidden variable or *daivam* showing a new direction to the harassed spirit can be gained. It is, therefore, necessary to find out what its instruments and its methods are? Tantra and its methods are known as the operation of *kriyāśakti* in the ancient Indian lore even as Yoga denotes the operation of *icchāśakti*. We have called these the formative power of thought and the directive power of consciousness. But what are these and how do they function?

14. The Sources of Energy

IN THE world today we speak of the sources of energy that get exhausted by indiscriminate use. Our civilization is fast moving towards this point of energy exhaustion, and we are told that once these sources get exhausted there is no way to replenish them. And so man is today in search of alternative sources of energy and, in this search, tapping the solar energy seems very much on the programme. But in the ultimate analysis it is man that is the user of energy. If the user of energy himself is enervated, then how will discovering new sources of energy help? Man must tap new sources of energy within himself before he sets on the journey of tapping new sources of energy outside. Julian Huxley, the eminent scientist, said in one of his articles:

> We must switch more and more of our scientific efforts from the exploration of outer space to that of inner space, the realm of our own minds, and the psycho-metabolic processes at work in it. It is here that greatest discoveries will be made, here that the largest and the most fruitful territories await our occupancy. All branches of science and learning can joint in the great venture of exploration.

There are the inner sources of energy which never get exhausted, for these are renewable sources of energy. In this book, we are not concerned with the outer sources of energy. We may, however, note that all outer sources of energy are non-renewable. Once exhausted they are gone and are not amenable to replenishment. We are here concerned with the user of energy, and for this our main interest lies in the source of inner energy. And this source is ever renewable and, therefore, always at the disposal of man. It is the man, aware of the renewable inner energy, who will use the outer energy well, neither misuse it, nor over-use it. Here we are essentially concerned with man, for he, in the ultimate analysis, is the focal point in the whole problem of energy.

In discussing the question of energy, we generally speak of the mechanical, the electrical, the thermodynamic, the nuclear and such other forms of energy. But there is one form of energy which is mostly lost sight of. It is available all the time, it is cheapest and is ever renewable. This is the thought-energy, tremendously powerful and totally inexhaustible. It is with this energy that Tantra is primarily concerned.

The most noteworthy thing about Tantra is that it uses whatever is available for the purposes of energy-release. Tantra is essentially concerned with the problem of energy even as Yoga is concerned with the problem of direction. It uses thought-energy whose source is inexhaustible, because it is ever renewable. Strangely enough, it uses thought to transcend thought. With the help of the mind, it transcends the sphere of the mind.

How is this possible, since thought itself has its own inherent limitations? Does Tantra seek to sermount these limitations? Mind is the creator of difficulties and handicaps in the further movement of a spiritual aspirant. What happens to these obstacles? Tantra places before the spiritual aspirant a method and a discipline which is quite different from the otherwise accepted approaches. The traditional approach in spiritual disciplines is to resist and relentlessly fight these obstacles and impediments. Tantra has no truck with this way of resistence. Does it indicate the path of indulgence—indulgence in vices and weaknesses that stand in the way of one's onward movement? It speaks not of indulgence either. Neither resistence nor indulgence—that is the way indicate in the way of the Tantra. It is the third way which we have discussed in the earlier chapters. This is done by the use of the *kriyāśakti* to which we referred in the last chapter. We have called it the formative power of thought even as Yoga is described as the directive power of consciousness. We shall turn to the latter in subsequent chapters: here we are concerned with *kriyāśakti* or the formative power of thought, for that is the instrument employed by Tantra to deal with psycho-spiritual problems of man. Writing about these two powers, H.P. Blavatsky says in her *magnum opus*, *The Secret Doctrine*, as follows:

> Kriyāśakti—the myterious power of thought which enables it to produce externally perceptible phenomenal results by its own inherent energy. The ancients held that any idea will manifest itself externally if one's attention is deeply concentrated upon it. Similarly an intense volition will be followed by the desired result. A Yogi generally performs his wonders by means of Icchaśakti and Kriyaśakti.

If the utilization of these two powers is not in harmony, if their operations do not synchronize, then much harm can be caused and far more dangerous consequences may ensure than what happens by the misuse of nuclear powers. We shall come to this synchronization in subsequent chapters. Here we must concern ourselves with the possibilities enshrined in the use of Krīyā-śakti, the formative power of thought. Every thought creates an image or a form. If thought is desultory, then the form created is vague and weak too. But if thought is strong, then the form that it creates is also strong and vital. Thought is energy, far more potent than any form of energy with which man is familiar including the nuclear energy. Not only has it great potentiality, it is ever renewable. The greater the power of thought, the greater the beneficial result caused by it and aslo the greater the harm when misused. It is a great instrument for self-transformation, and it is also the means for self-degeneration.

We are initially interested in finding out the beneficial effects involved in the use of the formative power of thought we must say its conscious use for even otherwise whenever a person thinks there comes into existence in subtler realms of matter forms and images. But we are concerned with the conscious use of thought formations. We have said that it constitutes a powerful instrument for the processes of self-transformation. Now, in all acts of transformation there are involved two factors: (i) the pattern of behaviour and (ii) the quality of living. There are the processes of transformation and transmutation. The former implies modifications of behaviour patterns, while the latter is concerned with mutations, meaning the birth of a new quality of living. What is meant by the formative power of thought or *Kriyāśakti*? How does it operate? In modern scientific circles, more particularly in medical sciences, a word is very much in vogue, and that is visualization. However, this word does not convey the full import of the formative power of thought. Obviously, visualization is concerned only with the visual images or forms of thought. But in the formative power of thought it is not merely the visual aspect that is implied; the implication is that all the senses are involved in the formation of an image. Ordinarily, in our experiences we receive impacts of all the senses at the same time, for, as we have seen earlier, the human brain functions not in a digital fashion but more along the analogue functioning. A living image formed by the mind contains the impulses drawn from all the five senses, not just the visual impulses. That is why the word *kriyāśakti* is more appropriate than the word visualization. But since the word visualization is used today, we shall use it too, but meaning all the time the larger context of impulses received from all the senses and not just the visual one. The formative power of thought is extraordinarily potent as can be seen from the following words of Dr. Maxwel Maltz, an eminent plastic surgeon of America. He says in his book, *Psycho-Cybernetics*:

> Experimental and clinical psychologists have proved beyond a shadow of doubt that human nervous system cannot tell the difference between an actual experience and an experience imagined vividly and in detail.

If the human nervous system cannot make a difference between the two, then the brain would immediately start functioning with regard to the impacts that come from something imagined in the same way as it would do if something were actually happening. And so the power of thought, of *kriyāśakti* or visualization is immense. But this has relevance only to the modifications of behaviour patterns, and not the quality of living. It is out of the behaviour patterns that habit mechanism comes into existence. And habit is one of the major factors that brings into existence a closed system. We have discussed the subject of habit in an earlier chapter. Habit becomes a base for so-called security for the human mind, and so it clings to it, thus imparting rigidity to one's behaviour patterns. All transformations of a fundamental nature demand the system being rendered open and living. The first step towards it is the breaking down of the rigidity of habit mechanism. We are not yet talking about transmutation. But for transformation or modification, the rigidity of habit has to be eliminated. This implies changing behaviour patterns. Medical science today tells us that a person can move towards regaining health, only if he starts modifying behavour patterns. It is this which most people find difficult to do. We have seen earlier that before one comes to the positive experience of health, one must get rid of the symptoms of illness. It is a negative work, but it is necessary before the positive experience of health can be had. It is with the symptoms of illness that behaviour patterns are concerned. A change in behavour patterns is a precurser to the movement towards health. But the behaviour patterns rooted in habit-mechanism are not easy to dislodge. It is here that *kriyāśakti* or visualization is of great help. The instrument of visualization has tremendous possibilities. It has dangers too, but to this we will come later in our discussions in this book. It would be useful for us to have a brief look at the possibilities implied in the process of visualization before we turn actually to its technique.

These days we speak much about bio-feed processes. The method of bio-feed processes is to reconstruct those external conditions in which certain reactions are evoked in the functioning of human organism. It serves as an inducement to the reactive processes of the human organism. It is meant to stimulate the brain to respond in a manner in which it responded when certain conditions obtained in the existential conditions of a human being. We have evolved very sophisticated instruments for this bio-feed experiments. But we have an in-built bio-feed system in the form of visualization. It can create necessary conditions for the evocation of required responses. And the human nervous system does not see any difference between what actually happens and what is imagined vividly and in detail. This is a great possibility offered by *kriyāśakti*.

The brain is a computer, a bio-computer as it is rightly called. It functions far more efficiently than the man-made computers. Besides it is fashioned not along the digital but along the analogue system. Now every computer has to have a programme, and programme needs programming and a programmer. The same is the case with regard to the brain-computer. And it is here that *kriyāśakti* or visualization can be of very great help. Just as there is a language which the man-made computer follows, namely, the language of symbols, the human brain, too, follows a language. It is the language of forms and images. This is what the formative power of thought can supply when consciously used. It is the clear and unambiguous language of images which the brain computer wants for its work of processing. It is this which conscious visualization can provide.

Now, in the problem of the modification of habits, it is the clear-cut programme given to the brain which is of tremendous help. If the brain is given a clear programme of habit modification, then it processes this programme like any good computer. But the programme must be clear with no vagueness about it. Since brain makes no distinction between the actual and the imagined, the latter is regarded by it as actual and starts working on it. Give to the brain a clear and a living image of a new pattern of behaviour, it starts processing it and produces a new behaviour pattern for the brain. This has been proved by experiments, and anyone can experiment it upon himself by starting with simple patterns of behaviour and slowly proceeding to complicated and complex behaviour patterns. It is not by the use of will power that habits can be changed, for will is like a king who issues orders and directions, but is not expected to execute those orders. The work of executing such orders is the work of *kriyāśhakti* or the instrument of thought formation. While the programming is done by thought power, the programme is handled by the brain. But what about the Programmer ? We shall turn to it in later chapters, for the subject impinges upon the directive power of consciousness of *icchāśhakti*. Thus visualization is of immense value in the field of bio-feed process as in the modification of habits through the programme and the programming.

It is visualization which is of great aid in memory training too. One's memory can be greatly strengthened, if, instead of feeding memory with abstract ideas, one were to use the image mechanism. An idea put in image formation can be remembered more easily than one that is in terms of mere abstractions. As we have seen, the process of visualization helps in rendering a system open and, therefore, living. It breaks down all those factors which render a system closed and mechanistic. A closed system becomes rigid and, therefore, insensitive. It tends to impart to the system a rigidity.

It is visualization which makes a system flexible, and, therefore capable of drawing energy from the environment. In the United States of America, medical men have proved that a patient who is recovering from his illness can recover much faster if his hospital room faces trees and shrubs than one whose room faces a brick wall. The trees give energy, but it is only the flexible organism that can absorb this energy, and a man recovering from illness has a little less rigid system than the one who has closed himself behind an overconfidence of so-called healthful conditions. It has been noticed that the athlete very often dies young due to the closed systems by an arrogance of so-called health. In April 1984 issue of the prestigeous journal published from America called *Science* it was said :

> The patients with the tree view had shorter post-operative hospital stays had lesser negative evaluative comments from nurses, took fewer moderate and strong analgesic doses, and had slightly lower scores for minor post-surgical complications.

This is so because the illness through which the patients had to pass had rendered their systems less rigid and therefore, more open to the process of taking in more energy from the living objects such as trees and plants. But it is not necessary for one to go through the experience of illness in order to be able to absorb energy from the invironment. Without being ill, through *kriyā-śhakti* or visualization one can render one's system open and sensitive. We saw in earlier chapters that a living system is vulnerable and, therefore, fragile. Such a state of vulnerability can be created by the process of visualization, for it depends upon the programme that is passed on to the human brain. In any case, programming and programme are the secrets of visualization, particularly through modification in the functioning of habits. Habit modification is one of the great contributions of the visualization technique.

Mental telepathy is now one of the recognized extra-sensory phenomena in the researches of psychology and para-psychology. Years ago one socialist writer in America wrote a book entitled *Mental Radio* in which he described the experiments in telepathic communication. It is not merely a mind-to-mind communication, it is a communication where one person seeks to initiate brain activity in the other person through mind-to-mind dialogue. Here one has to realize that telepathic communication can become more effective, if the communication is done through the language of images. For image is the language of thought and not the usual language of words. And so through visualization telepathic communication can become most effective and very much more smooth and restful.

But the question is: how is this done? What is the energy that accomplishes it? How is this energy derived, and from where? We said earlier that Tantra is energy restorer, and Tantra uses the instrument of *krīyāśakti* or the formative power of thought. Does the power of thought break down barriers in energy restoration? If so, how does this happen? How does it open up the human oganism to fresh absorption of energy from the outer environment? This must be so, for the environment is the storehouse of inexhaustible and renewable energy. How does this happen? We must examine the technique of visualization a little more deeply.

15. The Turning Point

EVERY serious bodily illness is usually followed by a period of convalescence which serves as a turning point in the physical state of the patient. It is a turning point, because it is a state where illness has gone but the condition of health has not arrived. Neither illness nor health—that is the condition which exists in this period of convalescence. It is a very delicate state, because it may create conditions either of relapse or of full recovery. Now relapse or recovery will depend upon the closeness or openness of the system pertaining to the bodily or mental organism. In fact, as we have discussed in earlier chapters, body and mind, though different, are closely related one to the other. And we may say that the openness or the closeness refer to the body-mind syndrome. It is a near-equilibrium state. Of course, we are not here discussing the state of biological convalescence. We are concerned with a psychological state of convalescence. It refers to the turning point in one's psychological realm. This may be depression or anxiety or frustration or a feeling of total rejection by one's environment. It is a condition of being down and out. Such a state does come every now and then in the life of a human individual. Its causes may be many, but such a feeling does come. Usually, one seeks an escape out of this state. Very often the escape, these days, is sought through drugs—may be tranquillisers or may be narcotics. Whenever there is a run-down feeling one seeks an easy way of escape, so that for the time being one is free from the pressures of the disturbing conditions. If during the convalescent period, one resorts to this, then one is bound to move towards conditions of relapse or recurrence of the same malady. The way to recovery demands a different approach.

114

The run-down condition obviously denotes complete loss of energy. The way must be found for the renewal of energy—to tap new sources of energy, for if there is fresh energy, then that energy itself will find the way through the impasse. This is possible through the use of visualization. By and large, the experiences of life are associated with events. An experience indicates a condition surcharged with energy. We cannot think of experience without the presence of an event, whether physical or non-physical. An event evokes energy, for it is a challenge which must be met. The greater the impact of an event, the greater the feeling of challenge. And it is this awareness of a challenge which calls out energy, as otherwise the challenge would render one flat under its impact. But events are external to oneself and, therefore, one must wait for the outer conditions to change. One is unable to order these changes in the external conditions of life. One seems to be chained to the immobility of outer circumstances. We want change, but it does not come. Obviously, this apparent immobility of outer conditions is the case of one's boredom. And this very boredom becomes an instrument of a greater feeling of energy depletion. It is a vicious circle in which one is caught, particularly in the modern civilization. We demand more and more exciting inputs from outside, and this recurring encounter with excitement causes greater and greater depletion of energy. There must be a never-ending excitement from outside—it is not dissimilar to the addiction to drugs. It is said that, when a dog bites a man, it is no news; it is only when man bites a dog that one calls it news. A constant demand for excitement and more excitement is the unhealthy cry of men and women of the present-day civilization. Events must happen all the time causing greater and greater excitement. An excitement being a challenge calls out energy from within, and so one feels that one is living and not dead. But the events that cause excitement are obviously pleasant and enjoyable. The unpleasant event, though a challenge, causes depression and not elation. Such an event still more depletes one's energy and so is likely to induce one to feel depressed and, therefore, in need of more drugs or more ways of escape. A painful event fails to call out from within any feeling of involvement so far as the experiencer is concerned. Man does seek excitement but of an enjoyable nature, for in a state of enjoyment he feels more energetic. An escape through drugs is once again for having pleasant experiences, but, since they are the means of escape, such so-called pleasant experiences do not evoke a sense of involvement from the one who is addicted to drugs. He gets what he calls pleasant experiences, but they are of an engaging nature. And, therefore, he must run away from the work-a-day world into realms of fantasy and day-dreaming. Such a person is more and more incapable of dealing with the problems of life. In fact, during intervals between drug-taking he is morose and depressed and, therefore, terribly bored.

There is no doubt that man's experiences are associated with events. And since events are not under his control, he must wait for such events to turn up and when they do he clings to them, frantically struggling to stop them from once again disappearing. But since events cannot be held as they belong to the stream of life, every coming and going away of such events leaves the person more depressed and dejected. Without events how can there be happy experiences? And without these experiences life seems dull and drab. How is one to get out of this predicament? And this, indeed, is the burning problem for men and women of the present-day civilization. A continuous depletion of energy and no saving grace at all. Man is bored and dejected in the midst of all the allurements of the modern age. Is there a way out? What else can man do except to seek escape after escape, whether through drugs or through other ways such as traditional religious rituals or such other prescribed disciplines or through the pursuit of Tantric powers or development of psychic and para-normal faculties. In the modern age such escapes have become a legion. There has arisen a bumper crop of pseudo-spiritual teachers who are ready to provide many avenues of escape out of the conditions of boredom and, therefore, of psychological imbalances. But, then, what else can one do? Since pleasant experiences are associated with events and since events are not under the control of man, there does not seem to be any way other than escape, whether bad or so-called good. We have to understand that all escapes are demoralizing, for it makes a man less and less capable of facing the situations of life. We saw earlier that the mind of man functions along binary principle: one must fight against circumstances or else one must submit to their requirements. But both the paths have proved futile to enable a person to live joyous and creative living. And so the question of questions is: what is one to do? One needs energy to live in a meaningful way. From where is one to find it? It is true that happy and pleasant experiences evoke more energy from within oneself. But, then such experiences can be had only through appropriate events. One cannot have experiences in void. There has to be a base of events. Now here the process of *krīyāśakti* or visualization is of tremendous help. Brain scientists tell us that human nervous system does not see any difference between an actual event and one that is vividly and intensely imagined. One can visualize a happy and a pleasant event vividly and in great detail. This seems to give to the bodily organism an experience of fresh energy evoked by such visualized events.

It is true that depletion of energy takes place in time. With the passage of time, the principle of entropy seems to function with great severity. Events come and go in the duration of time. In time the event appears and also in time the event disappears. If only time would have a stop! But time never stops. In fact, when one wants time to stop it does not, and when one wants time to move on, it does not. In moments of pleasure we want time to stop, in moments of pain we want time to move on. But it does not. If only there could be a reversal of time process, one would regain the lost energy. And one does need energy to tackle the problems and challenges of life. And we have seen that experience is associated with event, an experience of having the fullness of energy depends upon the event. But event is taken away by time just when one needs it to stay. In this predicament, it is visualization that comes, indeed, to the help of man.

While discussing the nature of time, we said that one aspect of time is reversible. This is what we have called personal or psychological time, and it is this time that matters. In the matter of experience, it is immaterial whether one deals with something actual or with something that is imagined or visualized. By visualizing intensely and in detail one can call back the event. Time is linear but time is also cyclic; it is both reversible as well as irreversible. Through visualization one can deal with the cyclic nature of time. Nature functions in terms of cycles like the cycle of seasons, etc. The subhuman creatures are guided by the cycles of nature. But not so the man. For example, in matters of sex feelings animals function in terms of the cycles of nature. But man is not dependent upon the cycles of nature, he creates his own cycle. In these cycles man experiences the same joys and excitements as would be the case in cycles produced by nature. The event is visualized intensely, and the experience is felt by man. For him event and experience are closely related. And since the human nervous system makes no difference between the actual and the vividly imagined, the experience of joy and happiness seems to be at the beck and call of the human individual. This is something which an animal cannot have—it seems to be in the hands of man due to *kriyā-śakti* or the formative power of thought.

Human beings are for ever plagued by the problem of the depletion of energy. Where energy is dissipated there man has no inclination to enjoy anything. He is lost in the whirlpools of depression and dejection. He feels like one who is swept in the current of life, unable to stop the current and so he goes whither the current takes him. It is this which causes boredom and dejection. He becomes alien to the experiences of joy and happiness, he has in his life no kick of excitement. He wishes to step out of this condition but does not know how. But man can create the world of happy past events or joyous anticipated events of the future. He can manipulate past and future as he likes by the power of visualization. Man can regain lost energy by the visualization of events belonging to remembered or anticipated future. The imagined events would call out happy and joyous experiences. And it is a known fact that man feels more energetic in moments of happiness and excitement born of that happiness. Thus, the feeling of happiness is indicative of renewed energy, and feeling of happiness is associated with events. Since man can call out appropriate events through visualization, the regaining of energy need not pose to him an insurmountable problem.

But then questions arise: is not the remedy of regaining energy worse than the disease itself? Will not the man following this visualization technique for ever begin to live in a world of fantasy and day-dreaming? Will this not become another way of easy escape from the actualities of life? Will he not be alienated from the world in which he has to live? Will this not be another form of drug addiction? Under the slightest pretext he will escape into the alluring world of visualization, thus becoming a stranger to the work-a-day world.

This is, indeed, a very pertinent and intensely relevant question. Visualization can very well become an escape. This is a danger which lies in the practices of Tantra. It may be an escape into the world of fantasy or day-dreaming or it may be an escape into psychic adventurism such as is evident today in all attempts at developing *kuṇḍalinī*. Behind all these psychic adventurism there is an element of escapism, a running away from the actualities of life because of the boredom or because of the painful experiences they seem to offer. In other words, visualization, too, can become another process of drug addiction. Tantra lost its credibility, just because it failed to take notice of this unfortunate development out of the practice of its technique. Sometimes the following of Tantric technique is in order to develop psychic powers for their own sake. Power for the sake of power is dangerous whether this has relevance in the field of nuclear powers or psychic powers. The craze for this is being witnessed today very much in country after country due to the boredom which modern conditions bring by technological advances. After having found material plenty, the modern man, particularly in advanced countries, asks the question: what next? Technological advances have now failed to cause any excitement. And so excitement must be sought in other fields. And the field easily available today is the psychic field where the awakening of *kuṇḍalinī* is the latest allurement. And so whether the escape is done through addiction to drugs or through the development of psychic powers, just for the fun of it, makes no difference whatsoever. Today there are many meditation cults developing both in the East as well as the West to the end of supplying new excitements to men and women who are otherwise thoroughly bored and frustrated. In these practices, there is no prospect of regaining fresh energy; rather there is the prospect of frittering away whatever energy one is able to get. In fact, after these practices one is exactly where one was or one is in a worse condition so far as energy availability is concerned. But, then, what is the solution? It is true that energy is our biggest problem for dealing with the new challenges of life. What is one to do? With loss of energy one has no confidence to deal with the situations of life. A new source of energy must be tapped and that, too, without exposing oneself to fresh problems of energy loss. How? That is the question of questions.

Visualization is conscious and, therefore, controlled image building. This image building is with regard to objects with regard to events and situations. But the events are not in the flow of chronological time. They are in the area of psychological time. An event in chronological time does not stay, it moves on, it comes and goes. It is this constant mobility of the event which causes the problem of energy loss with its consequences of frustration and exhaustion. It is this which produces the problem of boredom resulting in seeking escape after escape either through drug addiction or other escapes which we have discussed in this chapter. In the flow of chronological time, events cannot be made to stay. But this inability of man to stay the movement of events has produced the condition of incomplete experiences. The event is over but the experience is not. But an experience without an event has no ground to exist. It is this predicament which is handled by visualization. We have seen that, for the human nervous system, there is no difference between an actual event or an imagined event. And the imagined event can stay as long as visualization continues. If one creates a pleasant and joyous visualized event, then it would generate new energy for the use of the human individual. Since it can stay, the individual naturally would get greatly interested in the visualized image of the pleasant event. It is this which has the demoralizing effect identical with the effect of drug addiction. One would like to use this visualized image as a means of escape into the world of fantasy and day-dreaming. He would refuse to come back to the world of actualities. And this is exactly what is happening in the world today, particularly among the younger generation. This is the reason why Tantra is being more and more sought after, for it offers an effective means of escape into the world of visualization.

But without visualization there is no other way of regaining energy so as to meet effectively the ever-increasing challenges of the modern world. Is there a saving grace in the operational activity of visualization, or has man to submit to this vicious circle?

There is a way if óne would care to understand the technique of visualization in a scientific manner. Visualization is a veritable science with its own technology. The creation of visualized image has nothing to do with the method that goes on in the modern world by the name Positive Thinking, although the visualized image that we are talking about demands the eschewal of all negative images. Even then it is not anywhere near the technique of positive thinking. Nor is visualized image akin to hypnotism, not even self-hypnotism, nor is it like auto-suggestion. The visualization technique that we are speaking about is totally different from all the other approaches mentioned above.

Ordinarily, as we have been discussing in this chapter, there is a completion of an event, but the experience thereof remains incomplete. This incomplete experience of the past is the hangovers which prevent us from meeting any fresh challenge of life with a totality of response. Any challenge, met incompletely, naturally leaves behind a residue. When the event moves on but the experience has not been completed, there comes into existence a residue in the psychological field of one's existence. And it is this residue which is the creator of tensions, strains and stresses as obstructing the way to creative and joyous living.

What then is the right technique of visualization which

abolishes the gap between event and experience, thus opening
the doors of living through which man can enter a new dimension of living enabling him to move in step with the movement
of life itself? But for this we must know the technique of
visualization.

16. The Ending of Experience

THERE is no doubt that man needs constant replenishment of energy to meet the challenges and impacts of life. When the challenge is not fully met, there comes into existence the disturbing factor of incomplete experiences, and these in turn create the further possibility of accumulating more and more incomplete experiences. As we have seen in earlier chapters, it is these that bring into existence psychological memory and the operation of personal time. But to meet a challenge of life fully requires energy. It needs to be noted that the challenge of life is ever new because of life being in a state of flux. And so a full encounter with a challenge requires a constant renewal of the mind. It is this renewal which indicates the process of energy replenishment. It is in the context of energy that we have been discussing the technique of visualization. It is this technique that enables one to recall pleasant and enjoyable experiences as and when required by reconstructing events that have gone and also those that are being eagerly anticipated. In other words, in this technique there takes place a reversal of time—not chronological, but psychological time. When an event is recreated, the experience associated with it also becomes alive. That which had gone has come back.

While this is possible and extremely helpful in regaining energy with which to meet the challenges of life, there is also a great danger involved in it. And that is the possibility of man living in the enjoyment of imagined events, thus running away from the actualities of life. A state of psychological alienation is bound to come into existence incapacitating the human individual from encountering the new challenges of life. All types of psychological aberrations are bound to ensue, such as split personality and psychological imbalance. This is so, because a person would tend to cling on to the imagined event and refuse to proceed further. Thus, there would happen a flight from reality. In our ordinary normal experiences, events come and go but since they have been met not fully but partially, they leave behind a residue obstructing man from coming to the state of full response to incoming challenges. This is, indeed, the deep-rooted psychological problem of modern man leading to all types of illnesses of a psychosomatic nature. This is due to non-synchronization of the event and the experience. But through the technique of visualization, which we are discussing, another possibility is likely to materialize. And that is the non-ending of experience. Thus, we move from the ending of event leaving the experience incomplete to a condition of non-ending of experience due to the holding on to the imagined event. There has to be the ending of experience associated with the imagined event, so that one does not get struck in the stagnant condition of the continuity of the imagined and visualized event. The unhealthy escape into the realms of non-reality must be ended. To move from the problem of the non-continuity of event to the non-ending of experience would only lead us from the frying pan to fire. And so the question is: how to end the experience associated with the arousal of the visualized event? If the experience ends, the event will wither away by itself, for it is the experience that keeps the event alive. But how to end this experience, the source of renewed energy to meet the challenges of life?

It is this which has been missed in the techniques of positive thinking as also in the techniques of auto-suggestion or in self-hypnosis. Here the imagined event is clung to, and that, too, tenaciously. One is told to hold on to the imagined or visualized condition. One must hold on to the image of health that one has built or whatever else may be the nature of that image. This tends to create new tensions. In visualization an image receives its sustenance from the act of experiencing. If one's experiencing shifts, than the event too, becomes wobbly. But if one is asked to hold on to the event without experience, then naturally a tension is built up. Here the emphasis is on holding the event, and not allowing it to waver. The event is not allowed to wither. This is also what happens in the act of repeating a *mantra*. The mere mechanical recitation of a *mantra* is bound to create a sense of dullness, and, therefore, the effect of *mantra* is greatly lessened. That is why Patañjali in his Yoga Aphorisms says: that alone is *japa* where there is recitation with experiencing, where the mind and the heart function together. In other words, there is not only the clear formulation but also experiencing. This is what one finds very often missing in the techniques of positive thinking and such other devices. In visualization there is not only a clear thought formation but also an intensity of feeling.

The act of holding on to the imagined event is almost like the act of not allowing the real event to move away which one normally does. We have discussed this earlier stating that there is a lack of synchronization in the event and the experience. In our normal life, an event ends but not the experience. The experience remains unfulfilled, but the event cannot be stayed. And so pile after pile of incomplete experience gets accumulated. But in the process of visualization or in the operation of the formative power of thought, there is a reversal of this happening; for here if the experience ends then the event, too, ends, for the event receives its nourishment from experiencing. When the experience ends, the event withers away thus creating a synchronization of the two—the event and the experience. There is no hang-over and, therefore, no problem of tensions caused by non-fulfilment or by the factor of incompleteness. This happens in the sphere of visualization but not in the processes of positive thinking or such other devices. In the latter the event is an imagined one, but there is an insistence on holding on to it. In actual life one strives to hold the event but it slips away. In these new devices the imagined event is prevented from withering away, and in this effort it loses its vitality because of an absence of experiencing. Even if the factor of experiencing is there, such an effort is tantamount to creating new avenues of escape, as discussed earlier. If the act of living is not to become stagnant, then there must be a flow of event and experience. There must be a change or modification of events. But if the imagined event is changed creating conditions of psychological non-fulfilment, then we are once again caught in the same game about which we have been discussing in this chapter—the factor of a lack of synchronicity. And synchronization is of the utmost importance. In visualization this is possible and essential. If the experience is ended, then the event, too, ends.

But how does the experience end in the state of visualization? We have stated earlier in our discussions that Yoga and Tantra must function together. Tantra is concerned with the creation of an event, a visualized event. When it is not related with Yoga, the tendency is to impart continuity to the imagined event and to see that it does not wither away. If Tantra is concerned with an imagined event, it is Yoga that addresses itself to the ending of the event. But, then, are they not working at cross-purposes? They may, but they should not. They can and must work together so that the creation and the ending of an event maintain a rhythm and a harmony. But how? For this we have to find out: how is the experience ended and when is it ended? The how and the when of the ending of experience is most essential, if psychological synchronicity is to be maintained.

We have already considered the question as to why the experience should be ended, for otherwise there will be a tendency to hold on to the visualized event or image, thus making it a focal point for escape into realms of fantasy and day-dreaming. And the imagined event exists so long as the nourishment through experience is given. But before we discuss the matter as to *how* the experience is to be ended, it is essential to find out as to *when* the experience should be ended.

We have seen that the purpose of visualization is to regain energy which is otherwise lost. By visualizing a happy and pleasant event, the enjoyable experience can be recaptured, and the recapturing of such experience is, indeed, the regaining of lost energy. Since this is the fact, the experience should be ended not when energy is ebbing but when it is at its highest tide. And so, at the moment of ending the experience, one is in possession of a high voltage of energy. It is this energy which will enable one to deal effectively with the challenges of life. And so, at the moment of highest energy, the experience should be ended. But ordinarily we seem to be acting in a totally contrary state. The ending process is, indeed, a process of giving up. But ordinarily when does one give up anything that has been pleasant?

In all so-called religious or spiritual disciplines the factor of giving up has a very important place. In fact, the act of giving up is regarded as the supreme endeavour. This is to be found in both the Eastern as well as Western religious tradition. But, by and large, this giving up is done in moments of disillusionment or during moments when one is fed up with any particular experience. In other words, a thing is given up when it no longer holds one's attention. Now this is the moment when one's energies are at a low ebb. Let us turn away as it ceases to attract—this is the feeling of one who gives up an object or a thing. In this condition man is obviously in a state when his energies are squeezed out. He is like a psychological skeleton, devoid of enthusiasm and energy. And this state is ordinarily called spiritual, for it is regarded as turning one's face away from the things of the world. It is at this moment that the so-called act of giving up takes place. It is this which is regarded as taking to *sannyāsa* or to renunciation. In this context, it would be well for us to look at the statement of one of the most eminent thinkers and philosophers of the modern age, J. Krishnamurti. In his London talks of 1965, he posed the following question: 'How does one come to a point where in the full enjoyment of something, one ends it? To drop or end an event or an object at the moment of full enjoyment—this is what is indicated by him. And this is, indeed, the cardinal principle of Tantra. When an event or an object is dropped, at the moment of highest enjoyment, the presence of energy in its greatest intensity is felt, and yet it is not locked up either in the event or in the object. It is free energy available to man for undertaking the stupendous spiritual energy. With the ending of experience, the event also ends in the field of visualization. Ordinarily, an event ends leaving one's experience unfulfilled. Now, in the technique of renunciation followed in almost all traditional approaches, one strives to end the object or the event, leaving behind a state of psychological incompleteness. We are not talking about that again; for we have discussed it in earlier pages. We are talking of psychological or visualized object or event or image. Our usual efforts are to give up the visualized object or event. This is the basis of our so-called spiritual diciplines. The object or event in this case is some weakness or vice or something that is regarded as undesirable for the spiritual journey. But it is the experience of most people that such an effort is utterly frustrating. One is not able to drop it, because its sustaining source, experience, remains intact. In the *Bhagavad Gītā*, Lord Kṛṣṇa says that the objects of sense move away from a person of spiritual discipline, but not the relish for them. It is the centre of relish which is the focal point of experience. Thus, the objects and events may move away but not the centre of experience. The centre of experience remains active as ever, even though the events and objects end. From the centre of relish other objects and events arise, and so the problem is to end the centre of relish, not relish in general but relish pertaining to particular objects and events.

But when must the centre of relish end? After rendering oneself utterly dry and lifeless? If one comes to such an incipient state, then the spiritual life to which one aspires to move will be a lifeless state devoid of strength and vitality. To live a spiritual life and yet be lifeless seems a contradiction in terms, and yet that is what one comes to by the so-called spiritual discipline ending the event but not ending the experience. In the state of visualization, event is dependent upon experience, and so it is the ending of experience, the centre of relish, that is fundamental, not the moving away from objects and events. The latter will wither away by themselves when the centre of relish explodes.

We have attempted all the time in our spiritual practices to shatter the object or the event. This may be vices and weaknesses or may be undesirable patterns of behaviour. We strive to change the patterns of behaviour, but all that we are able to achieve is to dress up the old patterns with newer clothes. And so the same problem persists, because the problem cannot be solved by ending the event or the object but the relish thereto. But when can the centre of relish be exploded? Has it to happen when one is down in the energy-trough or when one is at the peak of energy-functioning? If the former, then one will move about as a spiritual skeleton, devoid of vitality and vigour. The ending must happen at the peak of energy, if one's spiritual life has to have any meaning or purpose.

One has to realize that one lives not merely in the world of sense objects but also in the world of mind objects. The former is known in Hindu psychology as *vastu* or the objects in which the senses live and operate. But there is another word in Hindu psychology which is *viśaya* and it is called mind objects, a field in which mind moves. In fact, this can be called the product of the mind while the former is the product of nature. In visualization we are concerned with *viśaya* or the mind-object. The objects belonging to the sensorial field move away and as they move away the mind feels a sense of non-fulfilment. It wants the sense object to remain, to stay on, but it does not, creating a sense of psychological craving, asking for more and more of that sense object. Through visualization one tries to create a mind object which will not run away but stay as long as the act of visualization lasts. It is through the creation of the mind-object that recapturing of the event and the energy thereof is sought to be recaptured. It is this phenomenon of mind objects that we are discussing at present. We are concerned with ending the experience, because with its ending the event —imagined and visualized—would by itself end.

But when must this experience end? In traditional spiritual discipline, the effort is to move away from sense objects. There is a completely misconceived but largely prevalent idea that it is the senses that are the villain of the peace, and so they must be curbed and controlled, even suppressed as they tend to take man away from the spiritual path. It is out of this that the cults of self-mortification have come into existence. One must not give way to the senses, and so whatever is pleasant to the senses must be strictly avoided. But it is not realized that sense objects do not stay, they move away. In fact, it is this which is the problem of problems at the level of psychological non-fulfilment. One wants sense objects to stay so that one can have time to enjoy them. But they quickly pass on with the current of chronological time. It is mind that wants them to stay, for mind wants to linger so as to derive psychological satisfaction. It is in this effort that the sense objects are transformed into mind objects, the *vastu* changed into *viśaya*. One can hold on to mind objects, but one cannot do that with regard to sense objects. It is the mind which is the villain of the peace, and not the senses. And so curbing and controlling the senses is meaningless, at best this will result in becoming less and less sensitive to impacts of life.

The change of sense objects into mind objects is being constantly done by the ordinary process of thinking, for every thought creates its form, and the material for thought is derived from sense reports. But this is done consciously and intensely by conscious thought formation, by *krīyāśakti* or visualization. And this conscious formation is to the end that pleasant events of the past can be recaptured so as to experience the reversal of entropy or for regaining energy. If energy restoration is the purpose, then it is obvious that it should be ended at the point of highest enjoyment, for it is then that energy is at its great tide. To end experience at the point of low ebb has no meaning whatsoever. The experience gained through formative power of thought must end at the highest point of energy functioning. And so there is great truth in what J. Krishnamurti says when he poses the question: how does one reach the point when something is ended in the hour of highest enjoyment? It is from the point of enjoyment that the experience must be ended, and not at the point of exhaustion. This is so, because the energy regained must be used for certain meaningful purposes, as, otherwise, the regaining of energy serves no purpose at all. But the question is how is this to be done? How can enjoyment end at the moment of its greatest intensity? And so, while we have seen the why and the when of ending the experience, we must turn to the how of this ending, and it is this that brings us to the threshold of Yoga.

17. The Union with Oneself

THE Yoga systems, particularly in India, are many and varied. Each system has its own goal and its own method. But one can say without any danger of contradiction that Patañjali's approach to Yoga is most systematic, showing attempts to synthesize the various Yoga approaches which were existent during his time. Patañjali did not initiate a new system of Yoga, but his remarkable genius co-ordinated all the then exist-ing systems into a whole. It is hardly necessary to say that in the Hindu tradition Yoga is one of the approaches of philosophy. Among the six systems of philosophy, Yoga is the sixth or the last. Just as Tantra is a technique, Yoga is perceptive wisdom. Tantra can succeed only if the human organism, in all its aspects, is kept open. The aim of Yoga is to render human psychological system living and, therefore, open. This is made abundantly clear in the vary first aphorism of Yoga, enunciated by Patañjali. While describing what Yoga is, he says: ' [It is] the dissolution of all centres of reaction in the mind.' The word used is *vṛttis* meaning tendencies of the mind. This is some-times described as modifications of the mind. After all it is habit or the *vṛtti* that modifies the nature of the mind, that is why habit is called one's second nature. It is an acquired nature —a nature that is superimposed on the real nature of man. To free the mind of all such superimpositions is the purpose of Yoga. It is hardly necessary to say that it is the superimposition which renders human mind closed, and, therefore, rigid. Yoga shows the way to making the mind completely open and, there-fore, utterly flexible. What else could render human conscious-ness completely open than freeing the mind from all centres of habit? And this is exactly what Yoga indicates. It is only when the centres of habit are completely disintegrated that one can know oneself—one can be united with oneself.

The very meaning of the word Yoga is union, but the question is: union with what? It is usually said that it is union with Brahman, the Ultimate Reality. But where is this Reality? The Hindu spiritual tradition says that *ātman* and Brahman are not different; the individual soul and the universal spirit are not a duality; they are one, inseparably one. And so union with Brahman is, indeed, union with oneslf. But, then, are we separated from ourselves? If so, what are we as separate entities? And how can one come to the union with oneself? Patañjali says that, when the centres of habit or reaction are dissolved, the seer is established in his own nature; otherwise, the seer remains identified with the acquired tendencies of the mind. The goal and purpose of Yoga have nowhere been described so clearly as in the Yoga aphorisms of Patañjali. When the acquired tendencies of the mind are dissolved, psychological organism of man is rendered living and open, ready to respond to even the faintest whisper of the soul, ready to understand the secret of self-transformation. It is only in this open state that the organism can be endowed with tremendous energy, for it is now in touch with the inexhaustible source of energy which is life itself. But how and when does this miraculous touch take place?

We saw earlier, in the last chapter, that it is only when the experience is at the point of highest enjoyment that it must end so that tremendous energy is available to the organism with which to enter the state of transformation. But how is this to be done?

In Patañjali's Yoga system there are eight limbs—four outer and four inner. The four outer limbs are concerned with certain behaviour patterns. These are concerned with the modification of the patterns of behaviour. This is, indeed, the meaning of *yama* and *niyama*, the first two of the four outer limbs They are concerned with modifications of habit, negative as well as positive. In fact, the first four steps of Patañjal Yoga are within the province of Tantra, concerned as they are with the modifications of habit or modifications of the reactive tendencies. The modifications of behaviour patterns, which are habits or reactive tendencies, are amenable to the technique of visualization, the conscious use of the formative power of thought.

In the use of the formative power of thought, it has to be borne in mind that through this power the thought-forms or images that are created must be of a positive nature, not negative. But visualization is a technique which is often not clearly understood. Visualization is a science, and it must be used as a science.

The process of visualization has four main steps which are not quite understood in the visualization practices employed in modern medical treatment. These steps are: the conservation of energy, the creation of energy, the concentration of energy and the communication or transmission of energy. It has to be borne in mind that energy is the very base of visualization. The purpose is to have more energy to deal with situations of life. And so the first step in this process is the conservation of energy, that is, stopping further dispersal of energy. One must preserve whatever energy one has and see that no further unnecessary use of that energy is done. This requires a state of relaxation; it has to be relaxation at all levels, body as well as the mind. It is not suggested that one must employ various exercises for relaxation; in fact, exercise for relaxation is the negation of relaxation. One must find out how one can relax quietly and without effort. For such relaxation alone can be fruitful for the purposes of conservation of energy. One can relax listening to soft music or looking at nature's beauty or looking at a beautiful piece of art or whatever it may be. Each person must find out for himself or herself as to the best way of relaxing in a quiet manner. The state of relaxation is not a condition of sleep or a condition of dozing off. It is a state of quiet alertness where one is able to switch on and off one's consciousness without any strain or tension. This is the starting point for all visualization technique. Very often, nay, most often, this is missed. This is gathering together of one's energy functioning. The point of relaxation is the focal point where one's energies are gathered, and not diffused in various areas of one's interest. It is after this relaxation, lasting for a while, that one must turn to the creation of fresh energy. This point, too, is very often missed in visualization practices for health or whatever it may be. Unless fresh energy is created, there is no chance of any visualization practice succeeding at all. We have seen that an event or an object which naturally awakens pleasant and happy feelings tends to generate fresh energy within oneself. And so, before attempting to employ visualization for specific purposes, there must be clear and intense visualization of happy events or pleasant objects. With this will come the recapturing of pleasant experiences as we have discussed earlier. When such release of fresh energy is experienced, one turns to the concentration of released energy. This concentration of energy requires the making of a clear and intense image of what one desires to have. This desired image has to be held for sometime, and it is obvious that only a pleasant image can be thus held. The image must not only be clear and vivid but also as detailed as possible, for this image is the programme which the mind will hand over to the bio-computer which the brain is for the purposes of processing. This programmed image is the visualization of something happy and pleasant. It does not matter what the subject matter of this image is—it may be concerning health and healing or it may be with regard to the resolution of any psycho-somatic situation. So there has to be the conservation of energy, the creation of energy and the concentration of energy. But that is not all, there has to be a communication or transmission of energy. This demands the letting go of the image that has been created and which has been the subject matter of concentration. In most visualization techniques, this letting go is completely absent. It is absent in positive thinking as well. And yet this letting go is the most important part of visualization technique, as important as the creation of the image. The letting go is equivalent to handing over a programme to the computer. If the programme is not handed over, what will the computer do, even the best computer?

And so handing over of the image-programme to the brain is essential in the visualization technique. For then only the desired result can ensue by the process of *kriyāśakti*, the formative power of thought. But it is this which is missing in all visualization experiments that are being pursued today. Transmission or communication of the image-instruction is possible only when after creation of energy and concentrating it on the desired programme (the image is mind's programme for the fulfilment of a particular theme) it is handed over to the brain which is the bio-computer. The computer is then able to produce a desired result, such result may be the modification of a particular habit or it may be the regaining of health. This handing over is equivalent to transmission or communication. In the very act of handing over, the work of the formative power of thought ends. In fact, this is the ending of experience about which we have been talking. And with the ending of experience, the imagined event also vanishes. This act of handing over the programme is described in Patañjali's Yoga Aphorisms as *pratyāhāra*, meaning withdrawal. But withdrawal of what and when? While defining *pratyāhāra* or withdrawal, Patañjali says: 'When senses imitate the mind in its act of withdrawal it is called *pratyāhāra*.' And so it is not the withdrawal of the senses, rather it is an imitation of the mind, meaning thereby that it is the mind that withdraws and then the senses follow. The senses move about in an event or an object, and it is the mind that experiences or enjoys. The withdrawal by the mind is the ending of experience even as the withdrawal of the senses is the end of the event. To attempt to withdraw the senses without the mind withdrawing is to get lost in the frustrating game which we have discussed. The event cannot subside so long as the mind is active in experiencing. And so the mind, the experiencer, must first withdraw and then the senses will automatically withdraw; for the senses by themselves never linger anywhere, it is the mind that makes the senses to do so. And so *pratyāhāra* is the ending of the experience, and the event which is in the field of the senses, too, will get eliminated.

We have said earlier that the first four steps of Yoga discipline advocated by Patañjali refer to Tantra and the last three refer to Yoga. It is *pratyāhāra* which is the meeting place of both Yoga and Tantra. In fact, *pratyāhāra* is the culminating point of Tantra, it is here that Tantra ends and Yoga begins.

The state of *pratyāhāra* is the point from where Tantra and Yoga bifurcate. From here Tantra moves on to the areas of psychic development, of the awakening of *kuṇḍalinī*, of the stimulation of *Cakras*, etc. By and large, the practices of Tantra have laid stress on this aspect, and that, too, without deeply examining the act of *pratyāhāra*. Without *pratyāhāra*, Tantra moves along the path of indulgence, and without it Yoga becomes a frustrating struggle against an object or an event.

Tantra without *pratyāhāra* becomes an act of indulgence even as Yoga without *pratyāhāra* becomes an exercise in fruitless resistence. And so *pratyāhāra* or withdrawal is the midpoint in spiritual journey. Mind, being the enjoyer, must end first before the object of enjoyment ends. Our usual efforts are in the direction of ending the object or the event; but it is the mind that must withdraw first, and then the ending of the object or the event poses no problem at all. What is meant by the withdrawal of the mind? A visualized image continues so long as mind's attention is focused there with the step of concentration which we have discussed. When the thought-attention is loosened, the image starts withering. It is the thought-attention which keeps the visualized image alive and kicking. It exists so long as thought is focused on it. But the thought-attention must be withdrawn at the height of enjoyment, and not during the moments of ebb, rather it must be during the moments of high tide. For it is only then that one has great energy to undertake the journey into the realms of Yoga. Yoga journey needs much energy, for it constitutes swimming against the current of life, for life as it is ordinarily lived has to be in tune with the demands of society and community.

In Hindu tradition there is a custom first to create an image of the deity to be worshipped, then the image is decorated with great pomp so that the devotee's attention is all focused and concentrated on the image. Then the image is immersed with great pomp. In fact, the immersion is done in a mood of great festivity; it is not done with any tinges of sadness, rather it is done with pomp and music, with great feeling of joy and exultation. This is symbolic of what we have been talking. The immersion, the dropping away, the withdrawal itself is not only a moment of festivity; the experience of festivity rises to its crescendo when the image is immersed. Here we see *pratyāhāra*

at the moment of highest enjoyment. This is, indeed, the culminating point of Tantra, and so from here ascent of Yoga begins.
It is Tantra that is associated with enjoyment even as Yoga is
associated with certain amount of detachment. Tantra denotes
the path of outgoing, the *Pravṛtti Marg*, as Yoga indicates the
way of turning inwards, the *Nivṛtti Marg*. These two must co-
exist so that there is withdrawal in outgoing, and enjoyment in
turning inwards. When they are together, as *Bhagavad Gītā*
says, there is no renunciation of action, but renunciation in
action. This is Yoga and Tantra together.

But how is the withdrawal to be done in the moment of
highest enjoyment? We live in a world of images. All our
actions and relationships are image to image. We even do not
know ourselves, we know only the image of ourselves. And
among the images the most obstinate, the real die-hard, is the
self-image. We have said that there has to be a union with oneself; in fact, that is the demand of true Yoga. But the question
is: have we been separated from ourselves? If so, what are we?
There is no doubt that our self-image has created a false perception of ourselves. It is only the self-image that we know. This
is what Patañjali called *asmita,* it is a sense of I-ness without
knowing the 'I'. For us the self-image is the 'I', and we are for
ever engaged in guarding and protecting it. Its continuity alone
is our life; its discontinuity is regarded as death, of which, we are
afraid. It is this, and all the other images that must go, if one
is to come to right perception. It is not a question of
substituting good images for bad. Every image, however noble
it may be prevents us from coming to right perception. In
visualization is the way of consciously modifying the image.
Here the image has to be not only clear and positive, but it must
be a living image, not a picture but a three-dimensional image,
one that can be touched or heard or seen just as a living thing
is experienced. The question is: if for right perception all images
have to go, then why take recourse to visualization where images
are consciously created? That is the way of Tantra—to use the
obstacle itself to transcend the very obstacle. In other words,
in the present context, it is using the image to transcend the
image. The image is the obstacle to right perception, and Tantra

says: use the image itself to transcend the realm of images so that one can come to right perception and, therefore, to right action.

We have said earlier in this chapter that one must transcend the image in the moment of highest enjoyment in one's play with the image. The playing about with the image is what we called a state of concentration of one's energy. How is this to be done? By eliminating the enjoyer from the act of enjoyment. The energy generated by enjoyment remains, but it is the user of that energy, the enjoyer that is sought to be eliminated. This process of eliminating the enjoyer is the act of *pratyāhāra* or withdrawal. This is the culminating point of Tantra, namely, to remove the enjoyer from the act of enjoyment. The act of enjoyment is at its intense height, and yet at that moment the enjoyer goes. We have said that *pratyāhāra* is the meeting place of Tantra and Yoga. At the height of enjoyment, the enjoyer is totally and completely eliminated. This is where the enjoyer must go—not earlier—for at the height of enjoyment one's energy is in a state of high tide. And it is with energy, in high tide, that the arduous spiritual journey for Yoga must be undertaken. With energy in low ebb the journey cannot proceed, one will fall back again and again for lack of energy. Then the journey will appear as a path of woe, somehow to be trodden but with constant and continuous setbacks. But how to remove the enjoyer at the height of enjoyment?

Surely, at the height of enjoyment there is no duality of the experiencer and the experienced, no duality of the observer and the observed. In that moment of intensity, if the enjoyer is active, then the act of enjoyment is broken up. And a broken-up experience always results in producing a hangover, a feeling of incompleteless or of non-fulfilment, and a non-fulfilled experience creates a craving which constitutes a desire for the continuity of that experience. Thus, here it is not the ending of experience. It is an interrupted experience seeking its fulfilment through change of events or objects. Here the problem is not solved, it is only shifted. At the height of enjoyment, and there alone, the ending of the experience can come into existence—leaving no desire for continuity in any form or behaviour. One goes through unbroken and uninterrupted experiences, one after the other, but each full and complete. A full and an intense experience admits of no duality of the perceiver and the perceived. With the ending of experience the event that awakened the experience also vanishes. And experience can be ended only at the height of enjoyment, and never in the moment of the ebbing of enjoyment. And it is this which Tantra has advocated all through the ages. It is the mistaken notion of Tantra that associated a complete experience with indulgence. In indulgence there is no ending, there is only continuity. The fullness of experience without indulgence has been the secret of Tantra. And it is at this point of the fullness of experience that Yoga takes over. The withdrawal at the hour of fullness is *pratyāhāra*. The withdrawal of the mind obviously results in the moving away of senses from sense objects as the senses normally do. But how is this to happen or as J. Krishnamurti says: how does one come to a point where, in the full enjoyment of a thing, the experience ends?

A broken experience or an interrupted experience is not a complete experience. In the intensity of experience, there is no duality, and it is obvious that the experience can be ended only in a state of non-duality. The very moment duality is born the experience is broken and, therefore, cannot reach the height of fullness. To end an experience at the height of enjoyment is to prevent the duality from coming into existence. When does duality come into existence? Obviously, this happens when the enjoyer enters the field of experience. And enjoyer is the thought, for it is with the entry of thought that duality comes into being. Thought is the creator of duality. And so, with the entry of thought, mind as an observer or as a perceiver begins to function. But when does thought enter? If the thought does not enter, then in the hour of the full enjoyment of the self-image, the image ends. And when self-image ends, the vision of one's true nature appears, one comes to the experience of being united with oneself. Another self-image may come, but once, one has known how to deal with the problem of self-image the coming up of such images causes no problem at all. In the moment of its coming it can get dissolved. But the question is how to prevent thought from entering the field of experience—whatever may be the nature of that experience, whether a self-image or a visualized event or object. There is no difference between an object, an event or a self-image, for all are products of visualization. How to end them in the moment of intense enjoyment?

Since it is with the entry of thought that the duality of the experiencer and the experienced comes into existence, one must see how and when thought enters the field of experience. If it is prevented from entering, then the experience will end at the moment of intense enjoyment. It is thought which demands continuity of an experience, which is pleasant and happy. And to demand a continuity for an experience is to sow the seeds of craving and a hankering. In fact, ending comes almost unconsciously—one is not aware that the experience has ended. In the moment of intensity, in the very act of enjoyment, there is an ending of the experience with no residue left. But for this the entry of thought must be prevented. But how? Once the thought has entered, nothing can be done. But if one can prevent its arrival—and that is the secret of *pratyāhāra*—then we will have enjoyment without the enjoyer. At the high tide of energy, there will be no user of energy. But without a user of energy what is the use of regaining energy? An entirely new user will come who will take charge of the restored energy; but in order to know who the new user is—one has to explore the field of Yoga. But before we discover the nature of the new user of energy, we must see that the old user is eliminated. The ending of the old is the field of Tantra, the discovery of new is the province of Yoga.

And so we must explore the moment of the arrival of thought, whereby the duality of perceiver and the perceived comes into existence. When does thought arise in the midst of experience? Surely, it arises when there is verbalization of the experience, whether articulate or inarticulate. It is not making an effort not to verbalize that is demanded, but observing the arrival of thought in the wake of verbalization. When thought arrives, there comes into being the duality of the perceiver and the perceived. And the perceiver holds on to the perceived. The experience cannot end, and its intensity is shattered to pieces.

Neither is there the ending of experience nor is there the fulfilment of experience. Patañjali says that the senses withdraw
from their objects or events in imitation of the withdrawal of
the mind. When there is visualization, clear and intense, but no
verbalization, there is the ending of experience at the moment
of highest enjoyment. The intensity of experience is not broken
for there is no arrival of thought, and so in that intensity itself
the experience ends, leaving no residue behind. The self-image,
the subject of visualization, lies shattered in the midst of full
enjoyment. The work of Tantra is over.

But how will verbalization end if no effort is made along that
line? It is not that the verbalization has to be stopped. What is
needed is just to watch its arrival, to hear its footsteps, just to
observe as it comes. But will a mere observation stop the act of
verbalization? This demands an investigation into the nature of
observation. If Tantra is the science of visualization, Yoga is
the art of observation. We must see what Yoga implies.

18. The Process of Self-Integration

IT IS our common experience that when, in the midst of enjoyment, one verbalizes, the intensity of that experience is broken. At the height of enjoyment there is a silence, not brought about, but one that has come naturally into existence. The experience may be witnessing the beauty of nature, or listening to exquisite music, or a communion in relationship. In fact, after a great event and the intensity of its experience, one does not indulge in talk, one silently walks away. As we saw in the last chapter, it is verbalization that brings into existence, a sense of duality. In the moment of intense experience, there is just the experiencing. In the act of experiencing there is neither the experiencer nor the experienced. And so, if in the midst of an intensity of experience there is no entry of thought, then, in the absence of a demand for continuity, the experience ends, and that, too, at the height of enjoyment. We were discussing in the last chapter as to how the arrival of thought can be prevented. It cannot be prevented, but its arrival can be observed. But is just an observation enough? Is the problem so simple? Can there be an ending of experience at the height of enjoyment by just watching the arrival of thought?

Verbalization is, indeed, the door through which thought invariably enters. And so it is there that its arrival can be detected. In this watching the mind has to be extraordinarily alert, and, yet completely choiceless. If one engages oneself in choice, then many intruders may pass unnoticed. In a choice, the mind is in conflict with what to choose and what not to choose. In such conflict naturally the act of observation is fragmented. As

142

we saw the practice of Tantra ends when there is the cessation of an experience at the height of enjoyment. But this ending implies the withdrawal of thought, for thought creates a sense of duality. The intensity of enjoyment breaks up with the entry of thought leaving the experience incomplete. And so at that moment the arrival of thought has to be watched. If after the withdrawal of the mind, there is an effort by thought to re-enter then, surely, the whole affair of withdrawal is nullified. And thought does attempt to re-enter in order to save itself from being debarred from playing its part in the process of experiencing. Thought for ever is interested in keeping an experience incomplete. And so up to the last it foils or tries to foil all attempts that lead to its death. And so the end of Tantra and the beginning of Yoga is a very critical moment. Either one is dragged towards indulgence or one is able to ascend into the heights denoted by Yoga. And so the watching of the arrival of thought becomes imperative at this critical point. This demands visualization without verbalization. And it is this critical point which opens the door to fundamental transformation.

We have discussed in the earlier part of this book the statements of the scientist, Prigogine, regarding order arising out of a crisis. Here we are talking of the critical point between the intensity of experience and the arrival of thought. In fact, this critical point lies between visualization and verbalization. The intense moment of visualization is the moment where the experience ends. But if at that moment thought enters, then the experience gets shattered giving birth to a sense of non-fulfilment. Then there can be no emergence of a new order. But if thought does not enter, then the energy released at the moment of intensity leads on along the path of a new dimension of living. To watch for the arrival of thought at the moment of intensity is to initiate a reversal of consciousness. It is this which leads on to the doorstep of Yoga. It is a crisis out of which either one moves towards total inertia or towards a breakthrough in a new order of existence. But what is the nature of this observation? This watching is a very delicate process. It is the first of the three inner steps about which Patañjali speaks in his Yoga aphorisms.

The word used by him is *dhāraṇā* which has been wrongly translated as concentration. The real meaning of the Sanskrit word is holding. This holding is not of an idea or the ideal which one is pursuing. It is the holding of the mind. It is holding the mind in a state of watchfulness. The mind ever watchful is the first of the three inner steps of Patañjali. The ideas may come and go, but the state of watchfulness remains uninterrupted. Usually, it is believed that concentration means not allowing a thought to move away but truly it is a state where the mind does not move away. One cannot hold an idea—ideas must come and go. But the state of *dhāraṇā* indicates that the mind is in a state of watchfulness, watching the movement of thoughts or ideas without any interruption whatsoever. *Dhāraṇā* is thus a state of watchfulness on the part of the mind. It is thus alone that the arrival of thought will be detected. In fact, the whole movement of thought will be detected in this state of watchfulness. This watchfulness is not of a watchman but of a witness. To see the movement of thought without any attempt to break it up— this is, indeed, the state of *dhāraṇā* the first step along the path of Yoga. This is what is indicated by the statement which we have introduced earlier, namely, visualization without verbalization. In the midst of the intensity of experience, there is no entry of thought through verbalization. Here in the experience there is no entry of thought through verbalization. Here the experience ends, a state where there is no entry of thought breaking up the experience. To watch without verbalization is standing on the threshold of Yoga. To watch the movement of thought without interrupting it, is really to enter the portal of Yoga. This is moving from *pratyāhāra* to *dhāraṇā*, the terms used by Patañjali.

About the three inner steps of *dhāraṇā*, *dhyān* and *samādhi*, usually translated as concentration, meditation and contemplation, Patañjali says that the three go together. In fact, the three are a unified whole, they cannot be broken up. It is impossible to say where concentration ends and meditation begins, or where meditation ends and contemplation begins. They together constitute the Yoga discipline, according to Patañjali; but they have no validity if not preceded by *pratyāhāra* about which we have discussed. Any step taken along the lines of meditation without going through *pratyāhāra* would be utterly meaningless. In *pratyāhāra* which we have dscribed as visualization without verbalization, one is able to regain lost energy. And one is urgently in need of fresh energy, if one is to undertake the arduous journey of spiritual life. One must enter the portal of meditation full of zest and possessing tremendous energy. The very first *mantra* of the first Veda, *Ṛg-Veda*, says: 'I invoke fire and place it in forefront.' Now fire denotes energy, and so the Veda says that energy is placed in the forefront, for one needs it on the arduous journey of spiritual life. And we have seen that when, in the midst of intense experience stimulated by vivid visualization, if there is no verbalization, then one is in possession of tremendous energy. It is a critical point where the anti-entropy principle seems to operate; it is, indeed, a point of the reversal of energy. After the critical moment, thought will surely come and must come. But the interval gives energy with which to undertake the observation of the movement of thought.

The observation of the movement of thought does require great energy, for it requires holding the mind. If it is the thought that has to be held, that would be a frustrating act. It is the mind that must be held, so that it can observe the movement of thought. To hold the mind which is for ever restless is an arduous task needing all the energy that one can call upon. And the energy is restored, as we have seen, in the split second when intense visualization does not embark upon an act of verbalization. In this split second the reversal of energy takes place. But then after that, the movement of thought will and must restart if visualization is not to degenerate into attempts at escapism. One must return to the world of the actual, so as to function in response to the challenges of life. But since visualization without verbalization is a moment of the reversal of energy process, one has the great advantage of being able to meet the challenges of life while in possession of great energy. And, in order to meet the challenges of life, there has to be an observation of the movement of thought which again requires the holding of the mind, of what Patañjali calls *dhāraṇā*. If *pratyāhāra* results in the restoration of energy, *dhāraṇa* demands clear observation of the flux and the flow of thought.

It is observation which is the key to real spiritual discipline. In Buddhism we find the meditative approach given in terms of what is known as *vipassana* which means special observation. The Lord Buddha said to his pupils that if they would follow the four-fold observation, then they would have nothing else to do, because that observation would give them the experience of *nirvāṇa*, of spiritual realization. One may ask: what is this special observation ?

We must see what the nature of our ordinary act of observation is. We have noted earlier the statement of a German physiologist who said that it is not the eye that sees, it is the mind that sees. In fact, in every act of observation three factors are involved: the senses, the brain and the mind. In the final analysis, it is the mind that must put its signature for finalizing an act of observation. And the observation of the mind is always selective. It blacks out that which it does not want to see. In other words, in mind's seeing there is always the factor of likes and dislikes. We have to remember that in the act of observation about which we are talking just now there is the observation of the flow and flux of thought. And its flow is very rapid; in fact, it is an incessant flow. It is idle to slow down thought but' what can be done is to slow down the mind. To watch the movement of thought, moving incessantly and rapidly, requires an extraordinary sense of awareness. If the mind is to be aware of the flow and flux of thought, then it must have an extraordinary capacity to see almost instantly. Ordinarily, a child observes almost instantly anything that is happening in the external world. Similarly, there must be an instantaneous perception of happenings in the internal world—that indeed is *dhāraṇā*. No selective awareness can do; and, therefore the special act of observation which we are discussing is extensive awareness, and not a selective one. To be aware of thoughts appearing from all the different areas of one's psychological field is what characterize extensive awareness. In fact, it means being aware of the flow of thought without any selection whatsoever. To observe without any interpretation or evaluation—that is what is indicated. For this the mind has to be extraordinarily steady. That is why we have stated that it is not the stopping of the thought current which is suggested but the steadiness of the mind, the observer. The great philosopher of India, Srī Śaṅkarācārya said in his well-known verses entitled 'Bhaja-Govindam' asking the pupil to 'do whatever he likes but in all that he did he must be aware, nay, he must be extensively aware of what he was doing'. This extensive awareness is the special observation about which we stated, the state of four-fold observation about which the Buddha said to his disciples. This is the secret of *dhāraṇā* or concentration as the word is ordinarily translated. It is not concentration on something, some idea or some thought, it is mind in a state of concentration watching without any interruption of the flow and the flux of thought. The unwavering mind observing the incessant movement of thought—that is, indeed, *dhāraṇā*.

General experience is that when one seeks to observe thought, it acts in a very shy manner. It shuts up its shop, and pulls down the shutters. This is mistaken as coming to a state where thoughts have been silenced. But this is not correct. It is a state where the thoughts have retired into their hiding places. It is not a condition where thoughts have been silenced, rather they have sought refuge in nooks and corners of the mind. They have to be sought out from their hiding places. The mind and thought are not identical. Thought is the activity of the mind—one of the activities of the mind. Mind is the producer of thought. In *dhāraṇā* one is asked to observe the activities of the mind, namely, thought, for mind is much elusive to seek out to start with. If one can observe the movement of thought keeping the mind steady, then thoughts would come to a silence, and it is only then that the mind which is thought-producer can be found. And so it is watching the movement of thought that is first demanded of the spiritual aspirant. We have said that *dhāraṇā* has to be preceded by *pratyāhāra*. And the latter is an act of withdrawal. H. P. Blavatsky in her '*Voice of the Silence*' says:

Withhold thy mind from all external objects, all external sights. Withhold internal images, lest on thy Soul light dark shadows they should cast.

Thou art now in *dhāraṇā*.

Thus *dhāraṇā* comes when in *pratyāhāra* the mind is withdrawn from external objects and internal images. This is the moment of enjoyment without the enjoyer. At this critical moment, if no verbalization takes place, then the experience ends at the height of energy-restoration. It is with this energy that one enters the field of *dhāraṇā* which is extensive observation of the movement of thought which starts after the culminating point of *pratyā-hāra*. This thought movement must start if one is to live in the world of the actual. The movement of thought can be observed only when it is in action—not when suppressed or pushed into its hiding places. Suppression of thought is not the silence of thought; in fact, in this condition it is seething and boiling in the hiding places to which it has for the time being retired. This happens when the mind is engaged in elective observation of the movement of thought. That is why we have stated that there has to be an extensive observation of thought and its movement. In selective observation the mind is motivated by likes and dis-likes. We have to remember that the mind is the observer, and thought is the object of observation. *Dhāraṇā* is mind's extensive observation. Here the mind is not sought to be eliminated; in fact, in *dhāraṇā* there is observation by the observer. All that the observer, which is the mind—is asked to do is to observe, that is, without restricting the field of observation.

What does the extensive field of observation mean? In all acts of observation, even the most physical, there are by and large two areas—they are the focal and the marginal. The focal is at the centre of the observation field, and the marginal is obviously in the margin whether to the left or the right of the focal area. In what is called concentration, the effort is made to focus one's attention on the area in front and making an effort to black out the margin. This is what we called selective obser-vation. And this is what is sought to be done in ordinary prac-tice of concentration. This creates tensions and strains, because it is not possible to get rid of the margin. To observe both the focal and the marginal activity of thought—that is what is indi-cated in *dhāraṇā*. This is what a driver of a car does all the time, his attention being in front which is the focal area, but he is also aware of what is happening in the margin to his left as well as his right. It is thus alone that the driver is able to drive the car with complete relaxation. This is what a musician or a dancer does, and this is what most people do when in the midst of noise and disturbance they remain glued to their work. Not to be aware of what goes on in the margin is to be dull and insensitive, totally unfit to go on the journey of Yoga. To be disturbed by what goes on in the margin is to show forth one's unreadiness to move on the spiritual path. To be aware of the marginal activity and yet not be deviated from one's movemen. along the way indicated by the focal direction—that is, indeed, the trait of *dhāraṇā*. This is, indeed, the nature of extensive awareness. This implies the widening of the perceptive view breaking down all factors that tend to make one narrow and restricted. In extensive awareness there is the widening of one's outlook.

Now the marginal area is not necessarily physical; in fact, we are here discussing the marginal area at the level of consciousness. It is hardly necessary to say that the focal attention is the awareness at the conscious level. At the conscious level, one is concerned naturally with the focal areas of awareness. But in one's life the focal awareness of the conscious mind is very greatly disturbed by what emerges from the subconscious mind. There is most of the time a conflict between the conscious and the subconscious states of consciousness. This is, indeed, the problem in the traditional practices of concentration. The conscious mind is most of the time engaged in pushing back the emerging factors of the subconscious mind. In the subconscious are the factors that have been suppressed; they are not always undesirable, but they are inconvenient to the conscious mind. Conscious mind seeks the way of success and so whatever seems to threaten the way of success is pushed down. And so the subconscious level is the storehouse of all the suppressed and pushed down factors of life. They are full of vitality and acquire greater vitality by virtue of their suppression. In terms of consciousness, they are the factors of the marginal area. The conscious mind is for ever engaged in resisting whatever arrives from the marginal areas of the subconscious. The focal and the marginal are not in alignment, in fact, they operate at cross-purposes. In the midst of this unceasing conflict, one employs the instrument of selective awareness, selecting whatever is conducive to the maintenance of one's respectability and one's movement towards social success. Here the mind is disturbed by the impulses coming from the subconscious areas. It is in this state that the mind must observe. Naturally, it cannot because of the constant fear of being overpowered by the impulses of the subconscious. Any observation out of fear is no observation at all. A selective observation is meaningless, for here one sees what one wants to see. There is no observation of what is, but only of what is projected. An observation where there is extensive awareness is alone true observation. Here the focal and the marginal are observed at the same time. There is no resistance, neither is there indulgence. At the physical level, one can understand extensive awareness as one in which the near and the distant are perceived together. But since we are talking of awareness at the psychological level, we have to understand this in terms of consciousness. And so an extensive awareness in this context would mean being aware of the happenings both at the conscious as well the subconscious levels together, at the same time. The mind that can see this movement of thought at these levels simultaneously has a steadiness of observation. Thought, it must be noted, is a reaction. We hardly, if ever, know what self-initiated thought is. All our thoughts are reactions to outer stimuli—the sensorial stimuli. When there is no outer stimuli, our thinking process lies in abeyance, almost in cold storage. When the sensorial stimuli comes, the centres of reaction are activized in the sphere of the mind and the thought process begins. The mind must observe this activity which happens in its own campus. Thought is the reactive process occurring in the sphere of the mind, while *dhāraṇā* is an act of observation by the mind of the reactive tendencies functioning within its own campus. But here the observation has to be of what happens at the focal level and also at the marginal level. Ordinarily, we resist the reactive tendencies of the subconscious levels of the mind. And these reactions, otherwise suppressed by the conscious mind, appear stealthily in dreams and symbols. When it is not allowed to come up normally, it comes in these dubious ways. Extensive awareness which *dhāraṇā* is indicates the way by which the marginal and the subconscious impulses are encouraged to come up openly, and not stealthily. And so *dhāraṇā* essentially means the establishment of a friendly relationship between the conscious and the subconscious layers of the mind. The conflict between the conscious and the subconscious cannot be ended unless the subconscious is persuaded to act freely and openly without indulging in subterfuges like dreams and symbols. It is only when this conflict is ended that one can move psychologically to a state of integration; while with the conflict raging all the time, one is bound to experience an inner and a psychological disintegration. The state of integration demands that the conscious and the subconscious levels function with absolute freedom and, therefore, without any fear whatsoever.

The free functioning of the conscious and the subconscious suggests the focal and the marginal areas operating without any interference from either side. It denotes a friendly alliance indicating trust and confidence in each other, resulting in a happy co-existence of the two. This is extensive awareness or *dhāraṇā* in the true sense of the term. Here no effort is made to stop the flow and flux of thought; on the contrary, it is an act of observing what emanates from the conscious as well as the subconscious layers of the mind. Here, there is no suppression of thought, nor is there any indulgence with regard to the thought process, the conscious and the subconscious act as friends, respecting each others movement with no interference at all. And so there is no need for thought to seek its hiding place, both the conscious and the subconscious are able to function openly, with no trace of fear on either side. The co-existence of the conscious and subconscious is, indeed, the secret of *dhāraṇā*, commonly known as concentration. Thus, all tensions are removed from the functioning areas of both. Here it is necessary to mention that not to be aware of the marginal thought-activity is to be dull and insensitive. To be aware and yet not to be disturbed is the key to the effective functioning of *dhāraṇā*. To be completely absorbed in the focal movement of thought, unaware of the marginal activity is not concentration. To have distraction and yet not to be disturbed is the essential quality of concentration or *dhāraṇā*.

It is only from this position that one can enter the field of meditation or the field of communion. It needs to be remembered that Yoga is a process, it is not an isolated event. It is a process of integration starting with *dhāraṇā* and moving through *dhyāna* leading up to Samādhi—these are the factors of the process of integration, namely, concentration, communion and communication. Not to know them as a process but as isolated and separate events is completely to misunderstand the way of Yoga. It is from the co-existence of the focal and the marginal and the establishment of a friendly relationship between the two that the act of observation can start. To create the necessary ground for this act of observation is, indeed, the work of *dhāraṇā*, it is laying the ground for extensive observation which *dhāraṇā* is. When in *dhāraṇā* the ground of the extensive awareness is established by the co-existence of the focal and the marginal, that intensive observation becomes possible. In the ground of extensive awareness laid by *dhāraṇā*, the prospect of intensive observation becomes possible. If the focal and the marginal can exist together on friendliest terms, then it is possible to watch the nuances of their relationship in proper perspective. This watching of the nuances of the relationship between the conscious and the subconscious is indeed, the basis of meditation. Thus, the three—*dhāraṇā*, *dhyāna* and *samādhi* constitute a process of self-integration.

The intensive observation is not opposed to extensive observation. In fact, it is observation in depth even as extensive observation is observation in extense. Intensive observation is not a selective observation, but something in depth. In other words, if extensive observation is by the observer, the intensive observation is observation without the observer. In extensive observation which we have called *dhāraṇā* there is the ending of the conflict between the focal and the marginal, between the conscious and the subconscious factors of one psychological being. But in *dhyāna*, the state of communion or meditation, one is concerned essentially with the elimination of the observer. There has to be a two-fold observation—the observation of thought and the observation of the thought-producer. But, in order that this observation may be effective, one has to follow the way of *dhāraṇā* where a friendly relationship is established between the focal and the marginal movements. With the co-existence of the two which is the basis of *dhāraṇā*, such observation of thought movement is possible. The observation of the observed and the observation of the observer are the twin processes that are included in *dhāraṇā* and *dhyāna*—the extensive and the intensive awareness of the movement of thought. The intensive is not the opposite of the extensive. In extensive observation, there is the widening of the area of observation whereas in the intensive observation there is the deepening awareness of the areas sought to be observed.

Yoga is not an event, it is a process. It is in this process that there comes the experience of integration. Integration is not a construct of the mind. In the state of integration one enters a new dimension of living. It is truly a fundamental transformation or psychological mutation. Patañjali says in 'Yoga Aphorisms': 'The birth of a new species occurs in the overflow of the stream of consciousness.' Thus there has to be an overflow in the field of consciousness. Now the overflow can stand no obstruction to its movement. It is in the act of observation, extensive as well as intensive, that the obstacles get removed. But observation is possible only if the thought process allows such observation to take place. If it shuts down its shop and pulls down the shutters, then no observation is possible. It is in *dhāraṇā* which is the coexistence of the focal and the marginal that necessary conditions are created wherein observation is possible. When observation is extensive, that is, when the focal and the marginal are allowed to coexist, then is one ready to embark upon the act of intensive observation. In *dhāraṇā* the two movements— the focal and the marginal—operate together moving in their own respective areas on terms where each respects the other and refrains from any interference. When this condition is brought about, then can a dialogue between the two become possible. If *dhāraṇā* is distraction without disturbance, *dhyāna* or meditation is the dialogue with the distractions. One is truly concentrated when one is aware of the distractions but is not disturbed by them. Distractions cause no disturbance, because they are allowed to function in their own sphere. The focal respects the margin and, therefore, the margin in turn respects the focal. Distraction without disturbance is, indeed, the nature of *dhāraṇā* or concentration. It is this state which naturally flows into the experience of *dhyāna* or communion. *Dhāraṇā* and *dhyāna* belong to the same process which leads to integration. We must explore what *dhyāna* is, we must know what meditation implies.

19. The Ground of Innocence

THE eminent thinker, Dr. S. Radhakrishnan, once said that the spiritual is not the extension of the moral, it belongs to a completely different dimension. Thus, there is a dimensional difference between morality and spirituality. But they are mostly regarded as identical. In morality, however, one is concerned with behaviour patterns. If one's life is in accordance with the socially acceptable patterns of behaviour, then one is regarded as a morally respectable person. But spirituality can never be measured in terms of morality, for it is fundamentally concerned with the being of man, not with the behaviour. The behaviour is a manifestation, and all manifestations are incomplete. It is the spiritual which is the whole, the moral is only a part. Besides, one's behaviour cannot be judged truly by patterns of action, one has to take note of the motives that underlie a behaviour pattern. Moral behaviour cannot be equated with social manners, it has to be infused with something much deeper. A truly moral person derives his strength from spiritual perceptions, otherwise his behaviour is no different from a polished man of society. What are these spiritual perceptions which become the motivating factors of a moral behaviour? Obviously, it is the perception of one's being, for that which arises out of one's being is truly moral. A mere moral change is a structural change, it is a surface modifcation. The consideration of the moral and the spiritual has much to do with what is commonly known as character building. Is character something that has to be built? In fact, character, in the true sense of the word, is a process of unfoldment. The unfoldment of one's being is, indeed, character. The *Bhagavad Gītā* used a very significant word to indicate this. It called it *svadharma*—that action which arises from one's being.

That is why the Gītā associated *svadharma* with *svabhāva*. The latter means one's own true nature. It says that whatever emerges from the ground of one's true nature is truly moral. In fact, a man of true character is rooted in his own true nature.

But the question arises: are there two natures, one true and the other not true? This, indeed, is the case, for there is a nature that is acquired. The true nature is identical with one's being. But we all build up an acquired nature—this is our defence mechanism. In order to survive in social environment we build an acquired nature which gives one social acceptability. One's acquired nature must be in accord with social norms and standards. And one is constantly engaged in this process of becoming where one has the assurance of social survival. There is becoming in all nature. But the process of becoming at the human level is completely different from the process of becoming that one sees in nature or in subhuman organisms. The becoming in nature is the expression and the manifestation of one's own being. And so in such becoming there are no elements of frustrations. One becomes what one is. But this is not so at the human level. At the human level the problem is not so much of a biological survival, as it is psychological. And the psychological survival is rooted in the operations of the human mind. It constitutes not the survival of the being but of the image that the mind has built. For man, therefore, the process of becoming is the process of the survival of the image. The image is the symbol of one's psychological survival. One may bring about some outer modifications in the image, but one is never willing to accept the breaking up of the image. In one of the Hindu scriptures, *Aṣṭāvakra Gītā* it is said by way of instruction by the teacher to the pupil: 'If only one would separate oneself from one's image, then would one experince Peace, Happiness and Liberation here and now, this very moment.' It is the image that hides our true nature from ourselves. To be united with oneself is to liquidate the image that one has formed of oneself. So long as the image remains, it is the image that functions. All our so-called actions are but the actions of the image. To guard and protect the image is the one concern of man as he lives. And it is this guarding and protecting of the image which has caused tensions and strains and stresses in one's

living. This factor of image protection has become greatly in-
tensified in the modern age becuase of the vast and the colossal
society that modern technology has created. It is a depersonali-
zed society where the human individual has lost his identity.
And so he must create an identity which gives him the sense of
being somebody in the otherwise non-identifying envoironment.
This false and fictitious identity is the formation of one's image
on whose survival alone man hopes to survive. The whole frustrating process which man all the time experiences is the becoming arising out of the demands of the image. Our becoming is the
product of the image, it is completely unrelated with one's being.
And the image is constantly threatened by social and external
forces. One has to be all the time alert lest our existence be wiped
off. And the image is like an iceberg; its tip that is seen is a very
small, tiny part of it; the major part of the iceberg is unseen,
for it is underneath. This is exactly the case of the image. The
image at the conscious level is just a tiny external, the major
part of the image is below the conscious level.

The entire process of becoming is impelled and motivated by the
image, not merely the tip of the image but the entire iceberg of
the image. Unless this image is shattered, there can never be the
vision of the being, the vision of one's true nature. And the image
has to be shattered again and again, for new images spring up
from the ruins of the old. As H. P. Blavatsky says: 'The mind is
like a mirror, it gathers dust while it reflects.' But how is the
image to be shattered? Who will do it? Is the destroyer of the
image other than the creator of the image? And if the destroyer
is identical with the creator of the image, how is one to deal with
this perplexing problem of the image? The images operate at the
conscious as well as the subconscious level. It is more difficult
to deal with the images of the conscious mind, because they are
surrounded by explanations, excuses and justifications, and so
they cannot be laid bare easily. They have to be dealt with only
after the subconscious images have been taken into account.
Surely, it is the conscious mind that will deal with the subconscious images. To deal with these images one has to explore the
way of *dhyāna* or meditation. During the earlier processes of
pratyāhāra and *dhāraṇā*, the ground has been prepared for

traversing the field of meditation. In *pratyāhāra* there takes place the energy release very much required for one's journey into the field of meditation. During *dhāraṇā*, a friendly relationship is established through extensive awareness, so that the focal and the marginal areas are not pitted one against the other. The margin is ready to talk with the focal and vice versa. It is in this background that the work of meditation starts. It is the work of total attention through both extensive and intensive awareness. In this act of attention, it is easy to observe the images that operate at the subconscious level first. For these images are comparatively external to the conscious mind. Obviously, it is easy to observe something that is external. Meditation is, indeed, the process of observation of, first, the external images, and then of the internal.

It is *dhāraṇā* that makes it easy for the mind to observe the images of the subconscious layers. In the background of friendly relationship established, the subconscious is willing to reveal its secrets. And if there is some reluctance on the part of the subconscious to do so, then the visualization technique would stimulate the subconscious to begin to speak and to reveal what it contains. It is true that, in the usual meditational practices, it is the subconscious that causes distractions by the images that it projects. These images cannot be suppressed because, by so doing they get stronger and, therefore, more troublesome. As we saw earlier, the subconscious shuts up its shop unwilling to reveal what it has. But because of *dhāraṇā* and because of the visualization technique used in the background of the work done by *dhāraṇa*, it is possible to make the subconscious reveal its secrets willingly and with ease. To observe these images released by the subconscious is the beginning of the process of *dhyāna* or meditation or communion. While defining *dhyāna*, Patañjali says in his 'Yoga Aphorisms' as follows: 'The uninterrupted stream of the contents of the mind is *dhyāna*. In other words, *dhyāna* is the observation of the stream of the contents of thought without causing any interruption to that stream. We have said it is establishing a dialogue between the conscious and the subconscious layers of the mind. When the dialogue tends to become dull and uninteresting, the visualization technique can be used to enliven it. But the conversation between the two must go on without any interruption. There is obviously an interruption when the conscious mind, in the course of conversations, passes its own judgements or does evaluations. When this is done, the old habit of the subconscious starts exhibiting itself, and this leads to its shutting up. But if the conscious mind observes the image-stream of the subconscious without any comments and stimulates it whenever necessary by the visualization technique, then the subconscious reveals its secrets with regard to the theme of meditation initiated by the conscious mind.

When the conscious mind observes the images revealed by the subconscious, the latter is gradually emptied of its contents. It is not an absolute emptying but relative—it is relative to the subject matter or the theme of meditation. And the subconscious naturally becomes silent when it has emptied itself. The external distraction gets subsided. There is no noise of the subconscious with reference to the subject of meditation.

While the subconscious has come to silence, it is once again a relative silence. It is silence with an object, for silence is with reference to the subject thought about. The external images have become silent, but still there are the internal images—the images of the conscious mind. How can the conscious mind look at its own images? It is like trying to look at one's own face. Surely, this is impossible. But if only the subconscious has become silent and the chattering of the conscious mind continues, then how can one come to the experience of meditation? For meditation is the discovery of the ground of innocence. For spiritual realization to be, there has to be the communion with the ground of innocence. There has to be a complete cessation of the pollution caused by the noise of the conscious as well as the subconscious mind. How is the ground of innocence to be touched, if the noise of the conscious mind does not cease? This demands an observation of the internal images—we say internal because they are cast by the conscious mind and we want the conscious mind to look at the images cast by itself. This is what we have called intensive awareness just as the observation by the conscious mind of the images cast by the subconscious mind is described as extensive awareness. It is extensive, because the focal and the marginal are both taken into account. It is more the observation of the marginal in the context of the focal. In this extensive awareness the focal by itself as not seen, or, if seen at all, it is only for giving a context and a perspective to the marginal images. It is truly for eliminating a conflict between the focal and the marginal. There is one point which needs to be borne in mind, and that is that the more clear the formulation of the focal field is the more pronounced and vital are the marginal images. If the formulation of the focal is weak and desultory, then the arousal of the marginal images will also be weak. And so, in the matter of observing the marginal images, the focal becomes an instrument. Since in meditation it is the focal that is regarded as vital, the disturbance arising in this area is greatly resented. In fact, this is the basic problem in all meditational practices. The focal problem can be dealt with first through its reflection in the marginal areas. One must first deal with the reflection before one deals with the real. And the marginal is the reflection of the focal, and like a mirror view the marginal shows something that is the opposite of the focal. Today physical science is talking of the Looking Glass Universe. There are many different and contradictory things that are being presented to us by modern science. It may be the view presented by David Bohm or by Sheldrake or by Prigogine or may be by other scientists. They are talking to us what is perceived through their looking glass. We live, indeed, in a Looking Glass Universe, for we see in the looking glass; and the looking glass shows what is placed in front of it. Thus, what we call the universe is what is seen from our point of view. The universe is seen from the framework of theory which we have formulated. What we see is regarded by us as real. What we call the universe is what is seen in our particular looking glass. In other words, there is great subjectivity in the so-called objective, perception of science. And with reference to subjective, there is nothing so subjective as the image that is cast by the mind. Among these images there is nothing more persistent and die-hard than the self-image. To regard the self-image as ourselves is to be caught in the same looking glass phenomena.

In the first stage of the meditational practice, one is concerned with the images of the subconscious which are regarded by
the conscious mind as external to itself and, therefore, easy to
observe. But, when it comes to observing the self-image and its
manifestations, one is naturally not on such a sure ground. As
we have said, it is like looking at one's own face. But, then, how
is this internal observation to be done? This is what we have
called intensive awareness. Can one ever look at one's face? Yes,
one can and that is in the mirror. We all have looked at our
faces in the mirror, and so we do recognize our faces. Similarly,
one can look at the self-image in the mirror of life, that is, in
the mirror of relationship. This relationship can be with reference to objects, persons and ideas. One can observe one's reactions to the three-fold areas of life's happenings. Such observation
would mean looking at one's self image. This is self-image in action, and true observation is possible only when self-image is in
the midst of action. It is interesting to note that self-image is very
shy; it is averse to having its mask removed. And self-image truly
is a mask. In fact, our daily existence is a masked existence. We
move about in life wearing different masks—as many masks as
life's situations demand. We are afraid of going about in life without
masks, for we do not want to be found out. If we are found out, then
that constitutes a great threat to our security and even our survival.
This wearing of masks for suitable occasions is moving about in life
with our self-image. This prevents us from living as we are but only
in terms of the acquired nature which the mask is. Meditation is
total attention to whatever life presents us with. But this attention is continually broken because of the demands and the projection of the mask. The continuance of the masked existence has
its demands, the fulfilment of which seems to be the guarantee
for one's safety and security. The mask or the self-image stands
in the way of total attention which meditation is. If extensive
wareness is the characteristic of *dhāraṇā*, it is totality of attention which is the hallmark of meditation or *dhyāna*. But how
can there be total attention when there is something all the time
obstructing the vision? And the obstruction is the self-image.

What does total attention mean? It means a clear, unobstructed perception of whatever one desires to perceive. As we

have seen, it is the image that stands in the way. How is one to get rid of these images, and above all the self-image? The image is the product of naming an object or a person or an idea. If anything is perceived without a name, then there is no obstruction. The name is, indeed, the obstruction. The name and the word are not identical, for the word denotes a factor of recognition while name signifies a factor of identification. Without the use of words one cannot exist in a society; in fact, one cannot communicate with each other. But we do not merely use words for communication, rather we communicate with names. The name is the identifying label, in fact, name is the symbol to locate a thing, a person or an idea in the realm of psychological memory. But can we see something, or experience anything without naming? Can we recognize but not identify? One must experiment with this in small events and experiences—looking at a tree, a flower, a bird, and an animal, a child—anything where no psychological invlovement, or very little of it, exists. In other words, if we can observe neutral, things and objects without naming or without verbalization, then that very process will enable us to flow into deeply psychological experiences without naming or verbalization. We saw earlier' that an experience peters out when verbalization or naming takes place. The naming is the entry of thought in the act of experiencing, and thought by its entry pollutes everything. Nothing remains innocent when thought has entered. If meditation is the discovery of the ground of innocence, then it must know experience without naming or without verbalization. The ground of innocence is the ground of being, and being is untouched by thought. It is the entry of thought that corrupts, anything untouched by thought is pure and innocent. With the entry of thought, motivations comes in, and it is the motive which constitutes the corrupting influence. J. Krishnamurti speaks of passion without motive. Needless to say, it is when there is passion without motive that there emerges right action.

But self-image is filled with the motives of self-survival, of self defence. How is the self-image to go? It is very strange, but self-image dies of exposure. So long as it is not exposed, so long it may seem invincible. But the moment it is exposed, it disintegrates. And meditation is looking at the self-image in the mirror of life, the mirror of relationships, the mirror of daily actions. Self-image is an internal image but, in order to observe it the internal has to be made external. And this is what is sought to be done by seeing the internal in the mirror which obviously is external. If we can see ourselves as others see us, much of the self-image would get shattered. But to see the self-image for oneself in the mirror of life is to see its destruction. An exposure of the self-image is its death. Another self-image may come into existence, but there is the interval between the death of the old and the birth of the new. It is this interval which is the moment of meditation. Meditation can never be continuous, it can be constant, meaning from moment to moment—not the chronological moment but the psychological. And the psychological moment is the negation of the self-image.

When the self-image is negated, even for a moment communion with what one is immediately takes place. It is union with oneself. And the experience of this moment, of this interval, is, indeed, the truly spiritual experience. In this interval lies the discovery of the ground of innocence. As the eminent writer, Carlos Castansida, says: 'The twilight is the door to the Unknown.' This interval between the death of the old self-image and the birth of the new is, indeed, the twilight in the realm of consciousness. It is there that the close circuit of the mind ends, and one is face to face with the new. The self-image is the ego, the 'I'— the centre which conditions all actions of the mind. When the centre is gone, the closed circumference, too, is no more. One is in the open, under the vast sky, with no protection. It is a state of vulnerability, and meditation is, indeed, a vulnerable state. This is the ground of innocence.

This ground is reached in total silence, not merely the silence of the external images but also the silence of the internal images— the silence of the self-image. But is silence the be all and end all of all spiritual endeavour? Is this not complete negation? It is silence that is not static, it is intensely dynamic. There is a movement in silence which alone is right action, all else is mere reaction. The ground of innocence initiates right action. But for this we must understand the dynamism of silence.

20. The Return of the Pilgrim

THE SPIRITUAL aspirant who went on his journey as a traveller returns home as a pilgrim. Such is the transformation that takes place in the course of his travels. And this transformation becomes possible because of the touch with the ground of innocence. The ground of innocence belongs to the land of silence. But it is a silence with its own dynamism. This silence is described by J. Krishnamurti as 'a movement in the mind'. And this movement comes into being when the movement of the mind ceases. There is a stillness caused by the cessation of the movement of the mind, both conscious as well as the subconscious. In the stillness exists a new dynamism—the dynamism called the movement in the mind. Who causes this movement? Surely, the entity that went on his spiritual journey is no more with the cessation of the movement of the mind. Then, who causes this new movement? It is the ground of innocence that initiates this new movement or it is the unknown that causes the movement in the mind. It is truly action without the actor. It is the unknown that is the cause of the new dynamism with which the pilgrim returns to his work-a-day world.

What will be the nature of his behaviour? Who can tell? In fact this was the question which Arjuna put to the Lord in the *Bhagavad Gītā* wherein he asked: 'What is the mark of him who is stable of mind, steadfast in contemplation, O Keśava, how doth the stable-minded talk, how doth he sit, how walk?' To this question of Arjuna, Lord Kṛṣṇa did not give any straight reply, because no reply can ever be given to this question. The spiritual life is not a life of imitation—life of morality can be, but not a life of spiritual perspectives. From the ground of innocence may arise many and varied patterns of behaviour, sometimes mutually contradictory. There can be no consistency about it —not that there is a conscious effort to be inconsistent. Consistency and symmetry are the virtues of the mind. From the ground of innocence may arise patterns of behaviour which cannot be put into any framework of the mind. They break down or rather overflow all patterns and codes of conduct. What arises from the ground of innocence has an element of overflow about it. And the overflow has tremendous vitality in it. The land over which the overflow moves is rendered rich and fertile just as what happens when the river overflows. The transformation that comes as a result of this overflow is most fundamental—it is, indeed, a mutation. In the overflow comes the richness imparted by the very source which we have called the ground of innocence. Meditation is, indeed, a communion with the ground of innocence which is the ground of being. All processes of becoming that emanate from this ground are not imbued with a craving for fulfilment, it is surcharged with the vital impulse of unfoldment. When becoming is for seeking fulfilment, then there is frustration. The becoming at the biological level breathes of no frustration, for it is fully and completely an act of unfoldment. It is the psychological becoming which has elements of frustration, for the search for fulfilment remains always insatiable. Here the process of becoming emerges from an idea or an ideal, a concept or a belief; and this constitutes not the ground of innocence, it is not the Ground of Being. Such becoming emerges from the background of thought—from the ground of the incomplete experiences of the past, from psychological memory. It is in the ground of being that there is a newness and a freshness, for there is no vestige of the past clinging to it. It is only this touch of the ground of being that brings about fundamental transformation; in fact, the secret of self-transformation lies in this communion with the ground of innocence or the ground of being. It is transformation without any seed brought from the past. It is the touch with the Ground of Being that implants a new seed in one's consciousness—not the seed of the past, nor of a psychological memory, but a new and a vital seed. Patañjali says in his 'Yoga Aphorism'; 'When there is a thinking with a centre, the impressions clinging to that centre will prevent new light from dawning upon human consciousness.' We very often say that we act from the centre, not merely from the circumference. But who has established that centre? Surely, it is the mind that has formed the centre. And, therefore, to it cling all the tendencies of the mind. The centre maintains the seed which has been the motivating factor of mind's activity. And even this centre must go, for it is the centre of mind's becoming. Patañjali says further while elaborating the idea presented in the above aphorism:

When the very centre of identity is destroyed, there is a complete cessation of all reactive tendencies, thus bringing into existence...an experience in which there is not even a thought-seed functioning as a centre.

The centre of identity is obviously the self-image. That is the ego or the 'I'. As long as this centre remains, no fundamental transformation is possible. But the 'I' cannot be destroyed by the 'I'—any effort by the ego to eliminate itself will only strengthen the ego itself—for the ego does everything with a motive, and its motive is to perpetuate itself. That is why the *Bhagavad Gītā* says that one can move away from sense objects, but what about the relish in them? This relish cannot be removed by the effort of the mind, for all efforts of the mind are motivated by continuing the relish in one form or the other. The *Gītā* says that the relish can go only when there is the touch of the transcendental. It is only when that which is beyond the mind is touched that the very centre of identity is demolished. But the question is: if this very centre gets demolished, then how does the pilgrim act? Or does he not act at all? If he does not act, then of what use has been his long and arduous spiritual journey? And if he acts, from where does he act? We have stated that it is the ground of innocence that acts, not the actor. But even this ground must have some centre from where to act. If the old centre is demolished, then does this ground bring into existence another centre from where to operate? Out of the ground of innocence comes into existence not a centre but a nucleus. A centre is static and, therefore, cannot contain the dynamic impulse of the ground. But a nucleus is itself dynamic, and it is through a nucleus that the ground or the unknown acts. And a nucleus gathers to itself more and more active cells through which to function.

This contact with the ground of innocence is what Patañjali calls *samādhi*—the nucleus for action. It is interesting to notice the way Patañjali has described *samādhi* or communication. J. Krishnamurti says: communion is communication. The moment there is communion the act of communication starts. Between communion and communication there is no time-lag—it is instantaneous. Communion is the experience of meditation, and communication is the nucleus of *samādhi*. Patañjali says: 'That truly is *samādhi* where the essence alone is seen without its form.' In other words, there is the perception of the formless freed from the prison-house of the form. To see the Formless is to see the Whole. It is in form that fragmentation takes place; the Formless is unfragmented and so the Whole. This perception is the culminating experience of meditation or *dhyāna*. And so this the ground of innocence. This verily is the void out of which fullness comes into existence. This is the being from which becoming, natural and spontaneous, emerges. The word *samādhi* really means the state of integration. In fact, one who has come to the experience of *samādhi* is an integrated person. It is this Integration which is the ground of being from where the process of becoming emerges.

The state of being is certainly the formless state. And it is out of the Formless that myriads of forms can come into existence. Hindu philosophy has described Brahman, the Ultimate Reality, as formless and, therefore, capable of millions of forms. It is formless in spite of its many forms. The many forms emanate naturally out of the state of the formless. The emergence of forms is the manifestation of the unmanifest. That which is essentially unmanifest reveals itself in myriads of forms. It alone can do so. The formless has no limits, but the form is limited. And so that which is formless has infinite forms. And the ground of being is formless, and so its process of becoming has no limit; it is smooth and spontaneous just as a flower blooms effortlessly.

How will the spiritual pilgrim act on his return? Who can say? It is something which belongs to the realm of the unpredictable. This is, indeed, the hidden variable about which modern science speaks. It comes, but its arrival demands the fulfilment of a precondition. And that is the cessation of the movement of the mind. The unknown enters the void of the mind. It enters only the ground of innocence. And its entry has such strength and vitality that it creates its own forms and expressions. With its entry, there comes a state of integration. It brings the secret of self-transformation with its entry. It creates a nucleus round which everything becomes integrated. There is a wholeness in which parts come together—they have not to be brought together. The dynamic nature of being brings its process of becoming—natural and spontaneous.

It is true that in this process of becoming, mind does come into existence; but it is different mind, a new mind, for without mind the experience of the void cannot be transmitted. It is true that communion is communication with no time-lag between the two. But communication is, by and large, non-verbal; it uses the language of symbols and gestures. But from the land of the symbols there must arise the language of words for the common man to understand. This language of words is the process of transmission. The spiritual experience must be transmitted if it is to create a new base and a new pattern for individual as well as social action. The *Bhagavad Gītā* enunciates a new principal of social action. It says that whatever authority of experience the superior man lays down that becomes the pointer along which others move. It is an authority of experience, not of scriptures nor of mere words. It is out of the experience of the ground of innocence that there emerges that authority of the superior man. This has strength and vitality not to be found in any other region. It is that which initiates a movement of social change. The secret of transformation discovered by the individual becomes the nucleus for a fundamental social transformation. The man of spirituality is not a freak, nor is he an unheritable mutation. Spiritual realization is a heritable mutation. Spirituality does not advocate the gospel of escapism. It espouses a scientific approach to social transformation. But for this there must be established a nucleus of transformation in the life of an individual. A nucleus is intensely potent and dynamic. The individual and the world are not two different and separate phenomena. They are one. The individual transformation is the beginning of a process which culminates in the fundamental transformation of the world. As J. Krishnamurti says: 'You are the world'. It is not that first the individual must be transformed and then he can undertake the transformation of the world. In the very transformation of the individual, the process of social transformation begins. It can never be halted, for the individual transformation finds its fulfilment in world transformation; it is an unbroken process.

In the return of the pilgrim is to be witnessed the beginning and the end of this process. What will be the nature of the new world that emerges out of this process? Its nature is upredictable. It is not a subject matter of mind's imaginative faculties. It may take whatever form it chooses. One thing is certain. Whatever be its form, it will breathe of integration and harmony. In the ground of innocence are seen the direction and the directive of a new individual and a new world.

Since communion is communication, meditation or the state of communion is itself *samādhi*—the true expression of the supreme void. We have seen that while Tantra denotes the formative power of thought, it is Yoga that indicates the directional power of consciousness. In the co-existence of the two lies the secret of self-transformation which brings into existence a nucleus of social transformation. In the co-existance of Tantra and Yoga we see this miracle of movement in the midst of stillness. The movement and stillness are not separate, one from the other. The movement is stillness and the stillness is movement, the wave is the particle and the particle is the wave. The secret of self-transformation is indicated by the Dancing Śiva in whose dance, movement and stillness exist together. In the Dance of Śiva, the Dance of Naṭarāja, lies the secret of self-transformation.

To see movement in stillness and stillness in movement is to come to the right perception of things. And perception is action; they are not separate, nothing can divide them. It is to see the non-existent in the existent, the unmanifest in the manifest, the implicate in the explicate. This is what one can express in the beautiful words of William Blake:

> To see a world in a grain of sand
> And heaven in a wild flower
> Hold infinity in the palm of the hand
> And eternity in an hour.

Or to quote the statement of the *Iśa-Upaniṣad*:

> That is Whole, this is Whole
> The Whole comes out of the Whole,
> Taking the Whole from the Whole, the
> Whole remains.

Indeed, it is in the perception of the Whole alone that the secret of self-transformation lies.

Select Bibliography

Bharati, Agehananda. *The Tantric Tradition*. B.I. Publications.

Blofeld, John. *The Tantric Mysticism of Tibet*. Causeway Books, U.S.A.

Bohm, David. *Wholeness and the Implicate Order*. Routledge and Kegan Paul.

Briggs & Peat. *Looking Glass Universe*. Fontana Paperbacks.

Campbell, Jeremy. *Grammatical Man*. Penguin Books.

Capra, F. *The Turning Point*. Simon and Schuster.

Colegrave, Sukia. *The Spirit of the Valley*. J.P. Trecher, U.S.A.

Davies, Paul. *God and the New Physics*. J.M. Dent & Sons, London.

Dossey, Larry. *Space, Time and Medicine*. Shambala.

Dreyfus, H.L. *What Computers Can't Do*. Harper & Row, U.S.A.

Fagg, Lawrence W. *Two Faces of Time*. The Theosophical Publishing House, Madras.

Fromm, Eric *et al. Zen Buddhism and Psycho-analysis*. Souvenir Press, U.S.A.

Gawain, Shakti. *Creative Visualisation*. Bantam Books.

Haman, Willis & Howard Rheingold. *Higher Creativity*. Jeremy P. Tarcher, Inc., U.S.A.

Hardy, Alister. *The Biology of God*. Jonathan Cape.

Jones, Roger. *Physics as Metaphor*. Abacus, London.

King Serge. *Imagineering for Health*. The Theosophical Publishing House, Adyar, Madras, India.

Krishna, Gopi. *Higher Consciousness*. D.B. Taraporewala, Bombay.

———. *Kundalini*. Shambala, U.S.A.

Krishnamurti, J. & David Bohm. *Ending of Time*. Victor Gollangs, London.

Mehta, Rohit. *The Creative Silence*. The Theosophical Publishing House, Madras.

———. *The Eternal Light*. The Theosophical Publishing House, Madras.

———. *The Fullness of the Void*. Motilal Banarsidass, Delhi.

———. *Krishnamurti and the Nameless Experience*. Motilal Banarsidass, Delhi.

———. *The Science of Meditation*. Motilal Banarsidass, Delhi.

———. *Yoga: The Art of Integration*. The Theosophical Publishing House, Madras.

Misra, Kamalakar. *The Significance of Tantrik Tradition.* Ardhanarishwar Publications, Varanasi, India.

Pandit, M.P. *Aurobindo on Tantra.* Dipti Publications, Madras.

Penfield, Wilder. *The Mystery of the Mind.* Princeton, New Jersey, U.S.A.

Prigogine, Ilya & Isabelle Stengers. *Order Out of Chaos.* Bantam Books, London.

Reincourt, A. de. *The Eye of Shiva.* Souvenir Press, England.

Russell, Peter. *The Awakening Earth.* Arc Paperbacks, London.

Siegel, Bernis S. *Love, Medicine and Miracles.* Harper & Row, U.S.A.

Silva, Jose. *The Silva Mind Control Method.* Pocket Books, New York, U.S.A.

Simonton, O. Carl. *Getting Well Again.* Bantam Books.

Singh, Thakur Jaideva. *Vijnanabhairava.* Motilal Banarsidass, Delhi.

Smith E. Lester. *Intelligence Came First.* The Theosophical Publishing House, Madras.

Soma, Bhikhu. *The Way of Mindfulness.* Vajirarama, Colombo, Sri Lanka.

Talbot, Michael. *Mysticism and the New Physics.* Routledge and Kegan Paul.

Thera, Nyanaponika. *The Power of Mindfulness.* Unity Press, California, U.S.A.

Thompson, R.L. *Mechanistic and Non-mechanistic Science.* Bala Books, New York, U.S.A.

Wayman, David. *Hypnosis.* Unwin Paperbacks, London.

Wilber, Ken; Ed. *Quantum Questions.* Shambala, London.

Withrow, G.J. *The Nature of Time.* Penguin Books.

Index